T0073581

ME VS. US

Also by Michael D. Stein

Fiction
Probabilities
The White Life
The Lynching Tree
In the Age of Love
This Room Is Yours
The Rape of the Muse

Nonfiction
The Lonely Patient: How We Experience Illness
The Addict: One Patient, One Doctor, One Year
Pained: Uncomfortable Conversations About the Public's Health
Broke: Patients Talk About Money with Their Doctor

MICHAEL D. STEIN

ME VS. US

a health divided

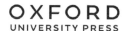

OXFORD
UNIVERSITY PRESS

OXFORD
UNIVERSITY PRESS

Oxford University Press is a department of the University of Oxford. It furthers
the University's objective of excellence in research, scholarship, and education
by publishing worldwide. Oxford is a registered trade mark of Oxford University
Press in the UK and certain other countries.

Published in the United States of America by Oxford University Press
198 Madison Avenue, New York, NY 10016, United States of America.

CIP data is on file at the Library of Congress

ISBN 978–0–19–763756–2

DOI: 10.1093/oso/9780197637562.001.0001

This material is not intended to be, and should not be considered, a substitute for medical or
other professional advice. Treatment for the conditions described in this material is highly
dependent on the individual circumstances. And, while this material is designed to offer
accurate information with respect to the subject matter covered and to be current as of the
time it was written, research and knowledge about medical and health issues is constantly
evolving and dose schedules for medications are being revised continually, with new side
effects recognized and accounted for regularly. Readers must therefore always check the
product information and clinical procedures with the most up-to-date published product
information and data sheets provided by the manufacturers and the most recent codes of
conduct and safety regulation. The publisher and the authors make no representations or
warranties to readers, express or implied, as to the accuracy or completeness of this material.
Without limiting the foregoing, the publisher and the authors make no representations or
warranties as to the accuracy or efficacy of the drug dosages mentioned in the material. The
authors and the publisher do not accept, and expressly disclaim, any responsibility for any
liability, loss, or risk that may be claimed or incurred as a consequence of the use and/or
application of any of the contents of this material.

1 3 5 7 9 8 6 4 2

Printed by Lakeside Book Company, United States of America

To Sandro Galea
Undaunted thinker, indispensable writer, attentive friend

To do for a community of people, whatever they need to have done, but cannot do, at all, or cannot, so well do, for themselves in their separate, and individual capacities.

—Abraham Lincoln on why government exists

It is surely far more difficult to form an informed opinion about what is good for society as a whole than it is to determine where one's self interest lies.

—Richard Posner

CONTENTS

ACKNOWLEDGMENTS

This project was helped along by the smarts and generosity of the faculty, staff, and students at the Boston University School of Public Health, where I have been fortunate to find a place to belong and to work for the past five glorious years. There, David Rosenbloom has taught me plenty, patiently answering my silly and basic questions as I tried to make sense of the beautiful mission of public health. Serving as Executive Editor of *Public Health Post*—our marvelous one-of-a-kind publication covering the health issues of the moment—for these five years and conferring with its dozens of writers has kept my mind carbonated.

Enormous gratitude goes to the team at Oxford University Press for their attention and care, in particular my editor, Sarah Humphreville, and Project Editor, Emma Hodgdon.

An extra thank you to my special reader and friend Peter Kramer for his finishing touches.

Toby, Alex, Sofia, Roy and Hester have made me so much better than I would have been without their love.

INTRODUCTION

With Health, as in the Rest of Life,
We Think in Terms of Me Not Us

Filmmakers understand the distinction between individuals and groups. When they shoot a character in a coma or receiving a bone marrow transplant, they know the viewer is thinking: she could be me. When they sweep across the debris of a village where an earthquake has killed thousands, they know the viewer, thinking on a different scale, may be moved and disturbed, but without any route for self-identification will be less riveted. For filmmakers, our collective reality is most comprehensible through individual life stories rather than large groups.

Similarly, our interest in health care, the medical care of individuals, supersedes our interest in public health, the well-being of collections of people. Medical care concerns itself with identifiable persons, whereas public health takes up statistical or anonymized lives, many lives seen through an extreme wide shot.

Let me offer two scenarios that demonstrate these two divergent perspectives.[1]

Scenario 1: You are the doctor seeing James, a 25-year-old man who rides a motorcycle and who has come to your medical

Me vs. Us. Michael D. Stein, Oxford University Press. © Oxford University Press 2022. DOI: 10.1093/oso/9780197637562.003.0001

office for a routine annual physical. At the end of his visit, you must make the choice between discussing organ donation or not bringing up the subject at all. Which would you do with James?

When imagining yourself *as the doctor* in this scenario, I believe that you would choose *not* to discuss donation. You would avoid this troubling issue because to bring it up is to move the conversation perhaps outside James' personal concern—he merely wanted the rash on his hand checked and a flu vaccine—and to turn what might have been a perfectly smooth and upbeat medical visit into an awkward occasion that includes an imagined and fatal accident.

> *Scenario 2*: Now approach the same question of organ donation imagining yourself as a regular, non-health care–employed citizen who lives in James' hometown.
>
> Young men who ride motorcycles are sometimes seen in medical offices for routine annual physicals. At such visits, the choice must be made between discussing organ donation or not bringing up the subject at all. What do you think doctors should do in these situations?

I believe that you would recommend that doctors, as a group, should discuss donation with these young men.

The first scenario introduces a medical question: How do I care for this patient? The second introduces a public health question: What should we want for our town? Medical doctors deal with one motorcyclist at a time, whereas public health-ers consider aggregates of young motorcycle drivers. If you gave discrepant answers (*I wouldn't* discuss donation in scenario 1, but every medical provider *should* discuss donation in scenario 2), it suggests that looking at a problem from different perspectives can change your judgment. The way you would treat *the unique patient* in front of you differs from the way you view *a group* of comparable patients. The physician is trained to be the perfect agent for each and every motorcycle rider. The public health practitioner, trying to come up with a policy, is trained to imagine herself as the protector of society, and considers a single patient as simply part of a collection of motorcycle riders. Discrepant answers suggest there is a conflict between these two perspectives.

We might admit that the public health perspective has a generous (though poignant) prospect—his donated organs could imaginably save the lives of others in his hometown if James has a fatal accident—but still, most of us would not insist that doctors and motorcycle-owning patients have this difficult conversation. We might agree with the group perspective and the public health interest in creating the largest possible base of transplantable organs, but we understand it is difficult to oblige doctors to follow in practice. And so, we would be hesitant to create and enforce a policy penalizing doctors if they did not discuss organ donation with motorcycle riders. Based on my informal surveys, persons who give discrepant answers to my two scenarios feel far more strongly about their "no" to the question in scenario 1 than about their "yes" to the question in scenario 2. We prefer and defer to the medical perspective; we naturally assume it.

Our fears about health have always been cleaved: Each of us worries about him- or herself (the *Me* perspective of medical health) *and* we worry about others (the *Us* perspective of public health). And yet, what is best for the individual may not be feasible for the group, and vice versa. Medical care and public health thus

3

represent distinct dispositions and attitudes, competing views of health.

* * *

The medical perspective turns on our powerful cultural ideas about individualism. Here in the first decades of the 21st century, we mostly think of life as an individual journey: You make your own career success or failure. You pursue advantage. You buy privacy. You are self-attentive, by nature, self-absorbed. The pursuit of happiness leads to a preoccupation with self. You live on the internet, the medium of self-presentation. You live for the moment. The ethos of self-help is ubiquitous; it dictates your view of health.

You manage small, daily bodily worries, believing most of the time that your health, your survival, is individually manageable. You live trapped in a single body, but you have high expectations for it. You want to control your body. You want to feel strong and healthy at all times. You expect bodily well-being and peace of mind. You embrace a therapeutic sensibility; every visit to the gym is full of dreams and plans; you can and will increase your balance, power, concentration; the triumph of the therapeutic is your salvation. All of this leads to the dominance of the medical perspective. You are a health optimizer, medically directed, driven by the latest medical studies. What matters is constant physical and psychic self-improvement. Psychic improvement means getting in touch with feelings, being authentic and spiritually awake. Physical improvement means having the perfect diet for your microbiome, the perfect mix of aerobic and strength fitness routines, waking up feeling rested, REM adjusted. You study the studies that show up daily on your newsfeed about how much to eat, exercise, and sleep. These are behaviors you control and that are life-preserving, the key ingredients of a healthy life, you've been taught.

Moreover, you believe nearly any person, properly motivated, can control his weight, how much she sits around, and how early he goes to bed. You hold to the belief that every individual has the wherewithal to make important life changes. It's a matter of will, of individual strength and perseverance; anyone can break, or better yet avoid, bad habits. Yet health problems related to the seeming lack of control of these "matters of will" are widespread; public discussion of stress and dieting is ubiquitous. Sure, you think, my neighbors may face obesity and diabetes and insomnia, but I can avoid these fates in my life by making the right choices, and by seeking treatment if and when I do get sick. Doctors can help; you turn to pills and procedures for optimization of the state of your health.

I am simplifying and exaggerating, of course. I am making us all sound like narcissists, infinitely pursuing immediate gratification and well-being. I do so in part to explain why, when we protected ourselves as imaginary doctors from the awkward organ donation conversation, I believe we were also unconsciously thinking of ourselves as the patient in the scenario. Not because we all own motorbikes or remember when we were 25-year-olds, but because when we go in for a physical exam, we do not want to be lectured about the risks of smoking or of being overweight or of not exercising, or, by extension, riding two-wheeled, tail-piped flamethrowers without a helmet. We want to be seen as ourselves, as individuals, not combined into a mass of at-risk men or women who smoke or are heavy or inactive. *My situation is unique,* we all think. *I don't care about some doctor's medical statistics about weight and illness and motorcycle accidents. Don't lump me into a group. I'm self-determined. I can defy all statistics.*

Whenever a doctor lectures us about our personal behaviors, that doctor is talking about our risk of *dying* if we continue our unhealthy activity. We don't like this threat; we prefer not to discuss it, just as we'd prefer not to discuss a fatal motorcycle accident in our future. In other words, we assumed a medical perspective in scenario 1 because we saw ourselves as patients, or potential patients.

We naturally think first in terms of doctors and/or patients and their needs in the immediacy of a health care setting. *I* do. I can't help myself; I am a doctor and I have a therapeutic sensibility. It is difficult to think into the future, a future of organ donation, or to think in terms of community, of what we could share with others, even in death. It is difficult, growing up in an individualistic culture, to think of ourselves as part of a group. Yet this is what a public health perspective asks of us.

* * *

If the medical perspective is one of independence, the public health perspective turns on the far less culturally accepted idea of interdependence. We contribute to and can respond to collective problems we actually see—traffic jams, polluted tap water, people asking for money at streetlights—as well as those that are mostly invisible to us: We all must clean up the mess left by the manufacture of nuclear weapons. But we can too easily look away. Our sense of identity is as consumers rather than citizens. Individually, I decide for and look after myself. Others usually come second, unless we are looking to blame. We watch people litter, but we don't pick it up. Unthinkingly, we coordinate when we agree to share roads, sewer systems, internet providers, fire departments. But those who object to the provision of food stamps wonder, Why should my hard-earned dollars go to feed anyone else? We are communal, but reluctantly. If that waiter has a cold, is coughing and sneezing, he should stay home, we think; but would we, if we needed the paycheck? Although more and more Americans live alone, we remain connected to other people: in buses on the way to work, at work, at school, through the air we breathe in restaurants. We can be indifferent to others' opinions of us, but we move through shared streets and shop in crowded stores.

To take a public health perspective is to admit that we live in a system of obligations and benefits. Private citizens become that mystery group "the public." Caring for others is a value, but not a certain one, even in a small group such as a family. If I am interdependent, my happiness depends on the happiness of those around me (substitute health for happiness).

The idea of "societal conditions"—poor sanitation, dangerous housing—as an explanation for why some became sick and some didn't was a 19th-century perspective, shaped by history and class and race. But this concept seems antique. Now sickness is up to each of us (and anyway we will be cared for by the medical profession) we believe, and vulnerability is a personal matter; preventing sickness, our collective protection, is a distant second thought. There's no parade because our water has become cleaner.

* * *

I have a friend who runs a hospital. She tells me about a patient who trips on a pothole, falls, and breaks his hip. The ambulance brings him to my friend's hospital. The doctors in the emergency room make sure that he—his heart and lungs—will be able to tolerate surgery. They take him to the operating room. They put a $20,000 piece of metal in his hip. They sew him up. They make sure he doesn't get pneumonia or a blood clot or a wound infection during his recovery period. They get him up and moving. They arrange for home services to keep him safe and ambulatory. They do all this expensive and expert medical and surgical work. And my friend asks me, in exasperation, "Now, who's going to fix the pothole? Does my hospital team have to go do that too?"

There has been a one-sided, indefatigable investment in health care. Health care and health are very different things. The pothole question sits at the intersection. Who is looking after public health? My friend's job is health care, she reminds me.

* * *

Let me give another example of these opposing health care and public health perspectives. Surveyed doctors agree that, if required by law, they *should* report to the motor vehicle department the names of patients who have seizures that might lead to loss of consciousness while driving. Removal of a dangerous driver from the road protects the public. But in practice, doctors *don't* make such reports to the motor vehicle department. Rather, they protect patients from losing their licenses; seizures while driving are rare events after all, and to strip away the ability to drive seems cruel. Again, doctors interact with individual patients in a way they would disapprove of if they were creating a public policy— the public health perspective—to keep the roads as safe as possible. Doctors take the individual patient or medical perspective because this is their oath.

Part of the issue is that we don't really like the word "should"—every medical provider *should* discuss donation; every doctor *should* report patients with seizures to the motor vehicle department. Should is an expectant verb that signals an obligation. We, and doctors, don't like to be told what to do, and we don't like general rules. We think in terms of unique cases and ourselves; we think less about the public good. We act by emotion—in this case trying not to upset the patient in front of us, or ourselves—while defending our actions and perspective as rational and consistent.

In the organ donation and the seizure report examples, is it contradictory to endorse one course of action in every individual instance and then reject it as a general practice? Can we treat a patient one way and groups of patients another way? Both can't be right.

* * *

Covid-19 presented the opportune time to discuss these Me and Us contending world views. In short order, everyone became a doctor, assumed an intimate perspective about health and disease transmission. It was all very personal. We cared about the health of individuals, those we loved. We listened for coughs, took temperatures. We monitored ourselves; we were medical detectives. We reconsidered underlying chronic conditions. We studied three-dimensional visualizations of lungs, the ground-glass images on X-rays. We learned how to wash our hands and judge which cleaning solutions killed viral particles, evaluated the filters of surgical masks. At the same time, we were engrossed by medical stories on cable news taking place in hospital corridors and intensive care units, and in the homes of relatives who couldn't be with loved ones in their last hours due to risk of infection. We were used to the viewing of medical drama depicted in too many prime-time television series. But we had never seen episodes in America about trying to prioritize limited gowns, about reusing protective masks. Now the panic was ours.

Covid-19 also made everyone into a health statistician, a public health aficionado. Each of us suddenly calculated the risk of our every interaction, with whom we spoke, what we touched, where we went, where we put down our shoes and groceries. We watched the case and death numbers on the television scoreboards mount. We counted and computed. We mapped fevers. We studied models. We named hot spots. We studied curves and inflection points, wanting new information about specific cities, counties, states. We thought about groups—over 65/under 65, preexisting conditions/no chronic illness. We were part of an aggregate, a pool of people a new virus was swimming through. Everyone became an epidemiologist—"epi" meaning above, "demos," the people; we sought an overview; we cared about the health of many, the health of populations. A public health perspective, virally focused, seemed a natural outgrowth of our observations and worries. Public health was no longer an abstraction (not merely a set of programs or a system we'd never really thought about); it became a story with a beginning, a middle, and, we hoped, an end.

During Covid-19, the competing Me and Us health perspectives were bridged by the let's-do-everything-we-can work of a pandemic. At first, medicine, always the dominant American mode, had few tools; doctors fell back on the methods of public health. Techniques used since the Middle Ages—quarantines, masks—were being resurrected in the age of artificial intelligence as our best short-term hope. But the investment in health care began immediately—clinical trials of antiviral and anti-inflammatory medications, the production of ventilators, our expensive belief in technology. Our old problems of medical insurance and who was paying for what tests arose. Our thinking returned to its medical mode, as we required help after we became sick. The bridge between the two perspectives soon started to buckle. The arrival of vaccines was considered a "medical miracle," but the uncontrolled spread of infection, Covid-19 was considered a "public health failure," a failure of infrastructure and trust, putting our unparalleled health care system at risk and the two perspectives at odds again.

Has the arrival of Covid-19 finally changed the way we think about public health and the historical divide between public health and medicine? For there to be permanent changes, we need to understand why it is we haven't sustained an interest in public health, despite so many opportunities to have done so. This returns us to the reasons we think primarily about others instead of ourselves only intermittently, only during and for a short time following a health crisis. We've seen this before: a spike in interest in our public health and common life (think of Hurricane Katrina, think of any mass shooting as we talk about community resilience and preventing *the next one*) followed by a fading away of concern. Civic responsibility, solidarity, shared goals matter to us during disaster—hurricanes, wildfires, maybe pandemics. But beyond crises, who are we responsible for? What are the limits? When you say "we," who do you mean? What's the widest community of which you spontaneously refer to as "we" or "us"? In our answer to that question lies the key to our future.[2]

I'm a primary care doctor, have been my entire working life. I signed up for, trained for, the medical perspective. I make decisions, lay down rules, give bad news. Each patient is gripped by emotion; in my office, they have limited time to speak and a lot to say. People expect to stay healthy and therefore sorrow is an inferno; no patient, no doctor is prepared for it. It's powerful and centers our attention on health on visits to doctors in their offices and hospitals. Recently I've come to fear that the medical perspective, the Me perspective—the individual matters most perspective—has become so prominent, so dominant in the way most of us think, we rarely consider the public health Us perspective. It is a disorienting idea that we are all connected; more natural is a belief in our separation from one another. The divide between medicine and public health may be unnecessary, but for now it exists. This misplaced emphasis on Me endangers us. It puts our health at risk because the solutions to our most concerning health crises, from obesity to climate change, will not come from self-concern or individual actions. We will need to resurrect and grow the Us perspective, and appreciate its unusual strengths. I have become a cheerleader for public health. And I think of my office practice differently now too, which I will come to later. Although doctors' offices are our least public space, the flesh of individuals adds up to a body politic as vulnerable as its weakest member.[3]

Before Covid-19, public health programs constituted only 2.5% of all health spending and the other 97.5% went to our health care and treatment system. Before Covid-19, the United States spent just $286 per person on public health but $11,000 per citizen per year on health care. The question is: Why such a discrepancy? And more important, if we'd spent more on public health, if we'd invested more in the preventive conditions of health—such as limiting poverty for a more equal economy, really trying to mitigate obesity—would we have been more prepared for Covid-19?

Covid-19 has shown us that discrepancies matter, and our population was vulnerable. Inequalities in wealth become inequalities in health.

The explanation, or rather the eight explanations, I and others have batted around for why public health has continually "lost" the perspectival conflict to health care, lost in our funding priorities and, before Covid-19, in our daily conversations, is the subject of this book. The restoration of the proper status of public health depends on our understanding of the eight reasons we have underestimated its value.

* * *

PART I

HEALTH DIVIDED

CHAPTER 1

WE ARE NOT SURE WHAT PUBLIC HEALTH IS

B efore Covid-19, I was reasonably sure from my conversation with friends that most people didn't know what public health really meant. Then suddenly "public health" was the vogue term, and everyone was talking about infectious disease prevention, and in particular, as our medical system was under threat of being overwhelmed, the failings with our existing public health methods. As Covid-19 erupted, when people used the phrase "public health efforts," they meant the remedies we had to deal with a surging pandemic *before* a person had to see a doctor—such as wearing face coverings or keeping a distance from strangers. A public health effort meant slowing the communication of Covid-19 from neighbor to neighbor. Once infections occurred and doctors were needed, the public health effort became a medical matter.

Our medical system would somehow have to handle the rush on emergency rooms, a tsunami that arrived on a predictable timeline after Covid-19 arrived in a city and filled hospital beds and intensive care units. If we "flattened the curve" of new cases, we could keep medical services available and give all people the care they required. (Flattening the curve also meant lowering the number of cases, in addition to spreading them out over time). We valued

Me vs. Us. Michael D. Stein, Oxford University Press. © Oxford University Press 2022.
DOI: 10.1093/oso/9780197637562.003.0002

medical services and their providers more than ever, although they were clinically limited at first, to our surprise and dismay, without an obvious treatment for a new coronavirus, and without a vaccine. Without a medical answer—and then even after vaccines arrived—an unceasing and contentious discussion of public health measures began, about differences between isolation and quarantine, contact tracing, safe spacing between people, and whether face masks were effective.

Yet even during the absolute worst periods of the pandemic, the major causes of preventable death were not viral; they were cardiovascular disease and cancer, with contributions from other common causes such as homicide and suicide and motor vehicle accidents. These were health challenges that we had not bought our way out of by spending $2 trillion per year on our health care system prior to Covid-19. If these were the leading killers, "public health" had to involve more than infectious disease prevention. Public health would need to explain how to engage with these causes of our static or declining national life expectancy—that is, after we manufactured a Covid-19 vaccine and tested novel treatments and our fear of the new virus had been reduced—for anyone to give public health its due and a larger share of the $2 trillion already committed to health. If dollars reflect societal interest, then understanding the reasons for the discrepancy between health care spending and the little we spend on public health had to be taken up again in the wake of our new interest in public health, so as to shift funding priorities and make us healthier, better, in the future.

* * *

Health care or medical care, medical science or medicine—I use these terms interchangeably because all refer to the same world view—focus on the causes of disease and the treatment of the individual (*Me*), by medication and procedure.

Public health, on the other hand, focuses on the causes of health. How can health be caused? Maybe a better way of saying this is by turning it around: Which life conditions and contexts (in concert with genetics and luck), when properly attended to, keep us well? Emphasis on the *Us*. Worldly conditions always apply to more than an individual.

Imagine a hula hoop on the ground. Imagine drawing a line away from the center at every point around the hoop so that the hoop has hair. If you set enough lines, you create a circle and can lift the hoop away. I like to think of the hoop as an individual. You could replace the original single hoop, any individual hoop, with a different colored hoop; either way, a public health perspective looks at the set of lines (the hundreds of conditions and contexts) creating the circles for every hoop.

*   *   *

The word *health* appeared around the year 1000 in Old English as "soundness of body; that condition in which its functions are duly and efficiently discharged" according to the *Oxford English Dictionary*. At that time, health was a divine responsibility associated not only with the physical functioning but also with mental and moral soundness and with spiritual salvation. Disease too was a supernatural phenomenon, often the consequence of sin.

A millennium later in the early 20th century, when the sciences of anatomy, bacteriology, and physiology were developing, health came to signify a disease-free state, based on the assumption that health and disease were distinct, objective, and observable phenomena. By focusing on specific diseases and their effects on specific parts of the body, this understanding of health neglected the individual as a whole. This thinking drew on a dichotomy: You were healthy or not healthy depending on if a part of you was diseased.

In the late 1940s, the World Health Organization (WHO), searching for a unique and universally valid definition, more holistically conceived of health as "a state of complete physical, mental and social well-being and not merely as the absence of disease or infirmity" (Constitution of the World Health Organization, 2020, 49th edition, p. 1). WHO was returning to the conception of 1,000 years before by defining health in terms of the presence of absolute and positive qualities.

By specifying both psychological and social dimensions, the authors of this early WHO concept of health acknowledged that health and illness are not merely physical but also include the capacity to complete certain tasks (get dressed or sing) and the ability to carry out societal roles (work as a teacher). The WHO concept shifted the focus from a strictly bodily perspective in which absence of illness was the sole criterion used to evaluate a person's status. Health must mean something more than un-diseased. But including the word "complete" implied a perfect state that was perhaps unrealistic and unreachable. If a person has a diagnosable condition—an objective, observable but minor skin abnormality such as eczema—is he still healthy? Would he be healthier without eczema? Does health only describe the maximal state? If so, it suggests that at a certain point the answer to the question,

"Could you be healthier?" is no. Yet at the same time, WHO introduced the idea of "well-being," which was broad and vague, hard to judge, difficult to apply in a precise way, odd to conceptualize as complete. The notion of well-being opened health to relativism, rather than maximization.

Social well-being necessarily includes an evaluation of functioning in one's environment. If health is to incorporate well-being, then healthy functioning indicates the capacity of a person to carry out their duties and responsibilities, and the ability to adjust to life stresses. So is maximal function (even if feeling sick) equivalent to maximal health? If a woman has lost a leg to bone cancer, has made adaptations and is not impaired or limited in that she performs all the social functions she ever wanted, can she still really be at a maximal state (when she's obviously not the same as she was before her cancer)? What is a handicap? Is a person born deaf healthy? If we don't investigate deafness, if we decide never to manufacture hearing aids, are we maximizing health? Is normal and adequate functioning a cultural construct? Will we need to conclude that what is considered healthy in one social context might not be in another?

We live inside bodies; we have roles in the world; we adapt. These three ideas seem to have a part in all definitions of health. "Not being sick," "feeling good," and "being able to do the desired and/ or required activities" seem like important elements. Well-being, or *wellness* as it became known, enlarges the definition of health by introducing the idea of quality of life: how to live happily, successfully, fruitfully. The broadest view of health not only would include these three basic premises but also would go beyond them by including self-fulfillment as a very relevant component of health.

Is this all more complicated than it needs to be? After all, we wake up sick—our joints ache, our eyeballs hurt; yesterday we were well; we intuit a binary categorization of health. Medical care is predicated on labeling individuals as sick or well. But is the risk of developing symptoms part of health? After all, some indicators of health are unseen, unfelt. A person who has a heart attack on Monday likely had substantial blockage to at least one coronary artery a day earlier on Sunday. We'd agree he was "sick" on Monday when his artery became acutely and completely blocked, but was he well on Sunday? How about if you were infected with coronavirus but have no symptoms—are you healthy?

Have these evolving definitions of health taken us to the conclusion that there are no clear distinctions between what constitutes health and un-health? Does health exist along a continuum within each person, judged over time—one day you can be healthier or less healthy than the day before—depending on how hard you look for trouble? Was health a look, a habit, a general condition?

Health allows you to do what you want to do to live a full, rich life, achieving whatever potential you wish to achieve. Health is a means, and perhaps not an end in itself. When I say "I'm healthy," it's personal. It's individual. This is a Me notion of health. We can probably agree on only two things, both Me-focused: Health is a consideration during every day of life; health comes to an end with death. But nowhere in this short history of the idea of (personal) health did I mention a guarantee of a long life as part of the definition.

What is the Us notion of health? What can we possibly mean when we say a public or population is healthy? The answer lies in the idea I introduced previously when I said that the diminishment of and the lack of funding for the public health perspective are leaving us *less healthy, less long-lived* as a nation. This equated the health of the nation with the longer lives (average life expectancy) of its citizens. Plural: citizens.

* * *

Each of us wants to feel healthy and to live a long time. Can we be in good health but have a short life expectancy? Yes. We can feel good and be able to do all the desired and required daily activities and yet have a suboptimal life expectancy if we ride a motorcycle, live in a violent neighborhood, smoke cigarettes, work right next to a bus depot, walk around considerably overweight, or don't have a lot of money. These conditions, these contexts and behaviors, on average, across a population increase the risk of dying prematurely. Of course, life expectancy is not something we feel or experience; it is not part of personal health; it exists outside the body.

The public health perspective introduces life expectancy as an average (as in: on average, growing up in your current zip code you are likely to have a shorter life span than if you lived in a zip code across the city). Life expectancy as an arithmetic term offers a view of the future that is very different from the health care perspective. No doctor in front of her patient is thinking, *This is how long people who have your life circumstances typically live.* Certainly, no doctor actually says anything like that to a patient because by doing so, she would be putting her patient into a group of similar patients, when all any patient wants to know is, How long will I live? Her patient doesn't want to know the average of a group. The doctor never says, "People who have your life circumstances . . ." because it robs her patient's uniqueness and she is trained to treat patients according to a one-by-one medical perspective. Instead, she leaves this view of health—*public, typical* health—to others.

The public health practitioner, on the other hand, doesn't look to measure the risk of any single person precisely but, rather, only the health of a population living in a community, on average, but with a clear eye on the range and full spectrum of health across community members. We understand that although we can forecast with reasonable accuracy the number of vehicle accidents each year throughout the entire country, individuals are never well represented by the average. We can't speak with certainty about the fate of any single person; we don't wake up in the morning knowing the chance that that day we will be in an accident. But unlike the physician, the public health practitioner believes we can get closer to answering, "How long will I live?" by recognizing that where and how we live and work matter. We see again how, according to the medical and public health perspectives, two concepts of health may be tied to different ways of measuring and thinking about the world.

One way to think about the distinction between medical and public health definitions of health is that from the medical perspective, health is a personal resource, something each of us calls upon to surmount obstacles and proceed in the world. You *use* your health to catch a bus, to have sex, to take on a new job, to take pleasure. You want *more* health not as a goal in itself but, rather, for what it allows you to do. Health is like energy, a force perhaps measurable in a person.

From a public health perspective, health is a collective resource, measurable only by counting across a population. The public's health can be determined year to year (infant mortality, cases of measles, obesity, life expectancy), is shared (unequally), and has causes, underpinnings.

* * *

The richest American men live 15 years longer than the poorest men; the highest income women live 10 years longer than the lowest income women.[1] This inequality is stunning, profound, disconcerting. And it's getting worse as the richest continue to make gains in life expectancy and the poorest fall back, widening the gap. Our first glance explanation for this statistic is that although rich people have the same diseases as poor people, if you are rich you get better medical care—better insurance, easier access to the best doctors, along with greater ability to pay for medications or procedures offered—and so survive longer. We move instinctively to a health care–centric, medical perspective. But does that check out?

Let's imagine that tomorrow we could eliminate cancer as a cause of death in the United States. This dramatic news comes as a result of the National Cancer Institute having devoted trillions of dollars to basic science research, and investors plowing money into companies that produced the new cancer treatments. The media fawned over every new development along the way with daily stories and magazine covers, and innovation awards were given to the newest medical heroes. Then, let's imagine that only the poorest people gained this benefit of never dying from cancer. Now, the Centers for Disease Control and Prevention estimates that the disappearance of cancer would increase average life expectancy by only a few years.[2] So in my example, take away one of the major killers in this country and the poorest among us still gain *only 3 years of life expectancy.*

Guaranteeing the poor would never get cancer only buys them 3 of the 15 years they need to catch up. Fifteen years is a vast difference, almost 20% of a lifetime. If we know that even a magnificent hypothetical breakthrough in medicine can add only 3 years to the poorest populations, how can we narrow the remaining 12-year gap? It's a critical question in the United States, and one that won't get answered through a medical approach, through the cure of a killer disease such as cancer or heart disease, or the provision of the best possible health care to every American. There are dramatic limits to the medical perspective, even as we make one-sided, indefatigable investments in health care.

In the same way that we devote enormous resources and effort and prestige to understanding the cures for cancers, we should likewise be thinking of how we might address this 15-year life span difference with the same energy and discussion and funding.

* * *

Yes, the poor are far less healthy than the rich. They smoke more, weigh more, exercise less, and have greater numbers of chronic illnesses. Chronic illness in turn reduces work and income; the poor grow unhealthier as they grow poorer. They are more likely to be uninsured, limiting access to care, compounding the hardship. It all adds up. The poorest 20% of Americans have a far lower life expectancy than the richest 20%.

This finding is true internationally and not specific to the United States. Yet lower income Americans are far less healthy than lower income Dutch or German or French or Scandinavian citizens and live shorter lives.[3] (Comparatively, the poor in the United States also have greater infant mortality, homicide rates, drug-related deaths, obesity, heart disease, and disability.)

Perhaps surprisingly, though, international comparisons don't look too good for upper income Americans either. When we directly compare the health of relatively advantaged Americans with their peers in other developed countries, we find again that Americans' health is worse. College-educated, insured, White, upper income Americans don't match the health or life expectancy of upper income strata Europeans.

We presume these insured and wealthy Americans receive adequate primary care, get access to medical specialists, and have the best chance at learning about advanced treatment options, so the difference is unlikely to be related to health care. Indeed, Americans older than age 85 years have longer life expectancies than Europeans, presumably because we spend a great deal more effort and money to extend life for the elderly. If you make it to age 85 years, you should be glad to be living in this country that spends trillions on health care annually.

But why American adults younger than age 85 years have a comparative health disadvantage compared to Europeans at every income level remains a mystery. For the highest income group, the availability of necessities such as food, housing, and transportation is not the explanation. Which life conditions and contexts matter, then, in keeping us healthy? Whatever they are, our health care investment has not been enough to catch up in life expectancy to the Europeans, even for the most fortunate among us.

* * *

I have set private (or individual) health in contradistinction to public health. But perhaps the opposite of public health is public suffering. Human (public) suffering can be measured and managed just like health. Researchers in the late 1980s created a global

Human Suffering Index that ranked countries on "life expectancy, daily caloric intake, clean drinking water, infant immunization, secondary school enrollment, gross national product per capita, the rate of inflation, communication technology, political freedom, and civil rights."[4] The developers were interested in asking, Are higher (worse) scores on the Human Suffering Index associated with greater population growth (which was thought to restrict economic and social progress for individuals and families as well as nations)? The answer is unclear, but if such a correlation existed, it would beg the question of causality: Does rising prosperity decrease suffering or does a decrease in suffering lead to greater affluence?

What's notable to me is that these researchers did not use the word "health" in their index of suffering, although one could imagine their list of the ingredients of suffering as approximating the boundaries and interests of public health. Of even greater note is that there's no mention of health care.

Keepers of the medical perspective would say: Yes, populations suffer from starvation. But can suffering be anything other than an individual experience? Individually, one can suffer more or less than a neighbor. For medical practitioners, alleviating people's pain is the first duty. Is a population suffering different from the sum of its sufferers? Is there an average suffering like there's an average life expectancy?

* * *

Whereas the medical perspective asks, "What can I do to make myself healthy?" public health asks, "What can we do to improve the health of others?"

By "health of others," do we mean that the measure of public health is simply life expectancy? Is public health a process of acting on behalf of equity, based on the knowledge that life expectancy remains inequitable? Then public health is a suite of policies, guidelines, unwritten laws, rules, procedures, and regulations that govern not only people's attitudes (racism, sexism) and behaviors (seat belts, speed limits) but also commonly held resources (clean air, water supplies) that play an outsized role in creating health.

What about conditions and contexts? If the world around us shapes our health, and our health is suboptimal, how do we reshape the world? Public health then must involve a set of institutions and transactions, programs and evaluative techniques, a method and an infrastructure.

If public health dictates eventual health care needs, then public health has an ethos of prevention, which carries with it a disposition, an attitude, a perspective, and some plans.

CHAPTER 2

IF PUBLIC HEALTH WORK IS PREVENTIVE, IT'S INVISIBLE AND BECOMES VISIBLE ONLY DURING CRISES

There's a metaphor I've found particularly useful when thinking about health. There are 11 players on a soccer team, with the goalie as the final line of defense.[1] The goalie in this metaphor is health care, the doctor. We certainly want a great goalie when we are sick. But by the time we need our great goalie, it is often too late. Better than asking our goalie for a miraculous save, we want to keep the attacking team (disease) away from our goalie to begin with. Most of the game is played by the other 10 players, out on the wider field. These players intermittently attack, but most of soccer is low scoring because more players are defenders. These 10 represent public health. They set the conditions for the outcome. They keep the game upfield and maximize our chances of winning, of staying healthy. In health terms, think of the field players as the water we drink, the air we breathe, our safety, our education, our social policies. Soccer is a game of prevention that depends on this group of 10, that is played with a We perspective.

Me vs. Us. Michael D. Stein, Oxford University Press. © Oxford University Press 2022.
DOI: 10.1093/oso/9780197637562.003.0003

The goalie, 1/11th of the team, is whom we rely on when we're not healthy. Health care, similarly, is only one part of the answer to health. But it's had a good publicity as the ultimate guardian of life and has concrete goods and services to sell—antibiotics and insulin and brilliant hip replacements. It certainly captures more than 1/11th of the resources and attention.

Metaphors are meant to create a shift in the way we think. I like metaphors. Hula hoops, soccer teams. I'll be using them a lot here.

* * *

"My health is influenced by your health," Lucas said to me in my first days working at a school of public health. Lucas is a colleague and beloved teacher at our school, an expert in how the U.S. health system compares to other countries' systems. From the first moment he heard I was a physician, he decided to orient me to the basics of public health; he figured I already had the medical perspective.

In some ways, his "My health is influenced by your health" statement is obviously correct. When I am sitting on a plane next to someone who can't stop coughing, I understand the statement in the narrowest way; I may be sick tomorrow because of my seatmate's pulmonary problem. But when I repeat Lucas' line to my family and friends, they don't really believe the statement more generally, beyond the example of airborne infectious diseases. They ask, "Does this mean I should be concerned with everyone's health and health behavior because it might eventually affect me?" "Come on," they say, "that's a lot to ask of me."

And then they have a friend who has a friend who was sitting in that bar, at that concert, in that office building working, in that synagogue or church or mosque, when the shots were fired. Dozens were wounded, some died, their friend's friend among them. Or they hear on the radio about the outbreak of measles affecting neighborhoods and towns, and about the million unvaccinated children, some of whom might be in their child's school. Or their neighbor's brother is killed by a drunk driver. They suddenly come face-to-face with the fact that we are all at the mercy of the behaviors of others.

And they come to one of two conclusions. One is fatalistic and inward-looking: Perhaps no place is safe for me. Their anxiety rises. They feel demoralized, uncertain, vulnerable. The other is more outward-looking: What can I do? What do we, as a society, need to pay attention to? How do we have a say in others' choices that touch our lives? Or, if not their choices, can we influence the effects of those choices, for their health and our own?

Infectious outbreaks and daily shootings and measles outbreaks impact the *public* health because they affect not just individual victims; families and communities and the public are changed too. Direct exposure to or even acquaintance with someone impacted by violence or disease is associated with *our* becoming depressed.[2,3] Being a witness threatens *our* mental health. Groups of people who don't know one another are at risk together in other health events. In a hurricane, I would want you to assist me if I was injured and vice versa. Many of us, if not all, will be affected by the health effects of global warming, our looming existential public health catastrophe. During these public health crises, we acutely realize that to think about ourselves, we also have to think about the lives of others. We see how we are connected. Health is a shared commodity—therefore I *should* be concerned, self-interestedly, with everyone's health and health behavior because it might eventually affect me.

A Me perspective that focuses on health care (sickness and cure) risks diminishing the Us perspective—your health influences mine—that is actually at play every day. But the Us perspective comes into clearest view during sinister acts that leave a community with mass casualties and during epidemics and uncontrollable acts of nature that bring on a different kind of panic. The split perspectives of individual health and public health have left us with a health divided.

* * *

"Our health is shaped by our shared social and economic context," Lucas continued a few days after I'd gotten settled. This was a few days after he'd told me, "My health is influenced by your health." I'd worked as a primary care doctor for 25 years, seeing patients one-by-one, a member of the health care sector that employed 16 million Americans, when I literally crossed the street from the hospital a few years ago and took this new job in a school of public health. I'd never heard Lucas' language before: our health. Academically, I'd walked across the street; philosophically, the distance was greater.

I knew where to go for *my* health—to a doctor's office, a clinic, a hospital. Bricks and mortar: These are the sites of an individual's health care. Where do *we* go for *our* health? Where are the sites of public health? Caring about *our* health is your new work, Lucas informed me. But where was the work of public health done?

Few people would know where to begin to find the practice sites of public health, and have certainly never visited one. If you started looking, as I did, by visiting your state's Department of Health in its generic office building with unopenable windows located on a side street somewhere in your state capital, you'd probably meet a guard at the front desk who would hand you a visitor's pass to stick on your coat, send you through a metal detector, and direct you to the elevators. You'd ride up three floors and step into a warren of masking tape-colored cubicles. The carpets need to be redone. The framed posters need updating. A government space, dusty and overheated and a little shabby.

Is this where public health is done? Is this where "our" health is shaped?

If this is where the work of public health gets done, who does it, and what is the work exactly? Health care is familiar; you would encounter matching emergency rooms in slightly different configurations in a hundred cities. If you went into any one, it would roughly be the same, as would the services. But the public health department in each of 50 states or 100 cities is unique and difficult to describe.

A medical visit has a structure, a pace, a time limit. There's the history-taking and the physical examination. There are only two people involved: one person searching for the problem; one person with the problem. The patient is the sole focus of attention; the patient knows when the visit starts and ends; there are prescriptions and recommendations. What is the rhythm and rallying point of public health?

I told Lucas that I'd visited the department of health and I'd talked to a few people there who'd described projects about lead in school drinking fountain water, a horse stable that was closed as a fire hazard, infections caused by a lack of sanitation at a liposuction facility, the monitoring of persons traveling from a country with a recent Ebola outbreak, and arsenic found in the dirt of a playground nearby. Lucas said, gnomically, "Public health is everywhere." And I said, "That's a problem. Everywhere is nowhere."

Public health is continually losing out to health care in the conversation of the public square (which also has no site, which is virtual, everywhere and nowhere) and in the court of public opinion (wherever that is) because health care is bought and sold, accessed at the time when we need it, whereas public health concerns itself with the visible and invisible dangers in the world and how we might avoid them when we might not even know they're there.

* * *

Americans believe strongly that we have an obligation to treat people who are ill. Which is why we put tremendous energy toward antiviral and immune-boosting treatment (the medical perspective) for the new illness Covid-19, initiating clinical trials we knew would take months to complete.

Conversely, we were slower to pursue testing for Covid-19, the determining of who was at risk, or contact tracing or quarantining, the low-technology centerpieces of prevention.

Perhaps we have less commitment to prevention because we valorize risk. Perhaps prevention implies restriction—stop smoking, lose weight, wear a mask—and we take pride in defying orders. For freedom, danger must be accepted. At casinos, we know there's a chance we can lose, which makes winning sweeter. I'm willing to take a risk even if you're not; rules—the cornerstone of prevention—shouldn't apply to Us; risk is a Me decision.

* * *

When Lucas first said, "My health is influenced by your health," I immediately thought: Wouldn't he rather pinpoint what, or who, puts him at risk personally? The problem is, he *can't* know. None of us can know.

There is the concept in health care of *universal precautions*. Health providers wear gloves when working with *every* patient because they don't know which patient might carry a bloodborne infection that is transmissible; the gloves are a layer of protection; they protect the patient too, who is unaware of which clinician might have an infection that can be transmitted. We can protect ourselves by staying away from everyone (not good for business) or by taking universal precautions. Personal protection while protecting others.

Public health is a form of universal precaution. That is, I have a personal stake in everyone's health and health behavior: Do you carry a gun? Were you vaccinated? Do you have infectious diarrhea when we share a public restroom? Covid-19 took this to an extreme: We couldn't expect to remain healthy unless we were all healthy; an infectious person arrived in town—we didn't know who this was, we couldn't know—and the cycle of new coronavirus infections spreading and decimating the non-immune began again.

Outside of a pandemic, we refuse to think that bad luck is coming our way. Toxic vaping fluid, contaminated drinking water, an *Escherichia coli*-on-lettuce outbreak—these problems will happen in other places and they will be reported on for a day or two, and we will read about them in the newspaper or hear a radio report perhaps, but nothing will happen to us or people we love. My health is not at risk, we think. We are able to put away our fear to a degree.

We have to put our fear away because otherwise we compound our worries beyond all reason. We are able to look ahead and then activate our great capacity for repression or we would be overwhelmed by the dangers of the world. We return to our diet, our exercise, our sleep, the Me domains we believe we can control. Meanwhile, the gears of public health work keep turning.

* * *

In 2014, the residents of city of Flint, Michigan, were drinking water that arrived from Lake Huron, until one day the city manager unilaterally decided to try to save money by using water from the Flint River, a waterway that had been a toxic industrial dump site for decades. The pipes newly opened from the Flint River delivered tap water that smelled bad, tasted worse, and ran brown and green in people's homes. Bacteria in the water soon led to a boiling alert and then the addition of decontamination chemicals. But that wasn't the end of it.

If the work of public health is invisible, often the target of its work is as well. What was invisible to Flint residents? Lead. Who had ever heard of lead in water? Lead was in paint chips scraped from old houses, not in water. In water, lead was colorless, odorless, invisible. Flint River water was innately corrosive, and the city had lead pipes that ran under the street, and water safety authorities were not adding anti-corrosion elements to the water as required by the Safe Drinking Water Act of 1972, so the river water leached more lead from the pipes. The inside plumbing of houses was lined with lead too. Flint is a poor city. Building age and poor housing conditions were most strongly correlated to those sites where lead levels were highest in the immediate aftermath of the water source switch.

Lead pipes had been outlawed in 1986 because lead is a neuro-toxin, causing irreversible brain damage, aggression, and a drop in IQ, memory, and attention in children. There is no safe bodily level. There is no antidote, no medical cure. The babies of Flint drank formula mixed with this water.

Where you spend your daily life influences your opportunities for healthy living. Our movement through our environment is a form of collective health care. Specific medical conditions—diabetes and depression, heart disease and substance use—can spring from the anxieties that diminish everyday life. These worries include the decision to send children to a struggling public school system or, with extra effort, to send them out of district; the heightened exposure to crime and blight; the diminished opportunities for finding healthy foods or other retail goods where no stores exist; the payment of high property taxes, and the receipt of poor public services in return. Water, one of our shared resources, now added to the stress of the primarily Black Flint residents. Water, used without a thought by most of us, affects the health of an entire population when it's unsafe to drink.

Only a wide view, the study of many patients, a population, allowed an onlooker to figure out what was happening to many of the kids of Flint who arrived one by one at doctors' offices around the city with odd behavior and headaches and anemia.[4] It took a whole city's worth of kids for concerned doctors to make the connection of symptoms with lead, a whole city's worth of blood tests to prove the association with the diversion of river water and overcome the denials of city officials.

Lead, an invisible poison, was introduced into the water supply at a moment of fiscal austerity by a city manager who made an out-of-sight policy decision in order to save money. For a low-income city with a declining infrastructure, this was particularly ruinous. Prevention is the work of public health, before you've heard there's a problem. But no one was watching for a problem in Flint; there was no monitoring after the water supply switch.

When the crisis arrived in Flint, after a year of investigation everyone starting talking about public health. Public health had been defunded in Flint; the city didn't have the staff to evaluate water safety or environmental or housing policies. But with the announcement of spiking blood lead levels in children, public health officials suddenly appeared in front of microphones, announcing bad news, making people scared and angry and upset, but also getting politicians to admit to the obscene failure of government for its Black citizens. In this case, if public health authorities had been asked about the water source switch, evaluated its effects immediately, and quietly demanded a reversal by the city manager, the preventive work of public would have stayed invisible. Instead, Flint has become a cautionary tale.

* * *

In Frank Capra's movie, *It's a Wonderful Life*, George Bailey, a banker on the verge of scandal, contemplates suicide on Christmas Eve. An angel, new to his prayer-driven work, with the unheroic name of Clarence Odbody, intercedes. Clarence shows George what the world would look like if he had never existed, the only sure way to measure the effect of our acts, a vision we can never get outside of books and films. The angel's depiction of a hideous future for George's friends, family, and town never comes to pass because George begs for his life back.

It's a Wonderful Life is the model for public health. "Terrible," Clarence suggests, "But could be worse." This is the hoped-for outcome of prevention. What might have been avoided in Flint. History is what happens, but the angel of alternate history tells us that we are making history all the time because of what *doesn't happen* as well as what does.[5] The Cherokee Nation shutting down 23% of the world's uranium production. Smallpox eliminated between 1967 and 1977. A nuclear waste dump that never existed; a road that wasn't cut through forest; a factory that didn't spew dioxin, nitrous oxide, or heavy metals. These environmental victories look like nothing happened; they give us places where there is nothing to see; they are triumphs of activism and the invisible.

Prevention *is* alternate history, plus a story of what we have done that kept the world from becoming worse. Like George with the help of his guardian angel, public health practitioners can help us see the atrocities *not* unfolding.

* * *

The early months of Covid-19 were all about predictions. Epidemiologists and economists made models—how transmissible the virus was, how many cases, how many deaths, how broad the economic downturn—and politicians displayed them in front of cameras.

In the midst of Covid-19, more than one prominent television commentator opined that social distancing measures had proven completely unnecessary. The basis for their conclusions was that fewer people had died than authorities said would die in the absence of stay-at-home orders. Therefore, they reasoned, the orders were unnecessary.

One such commentator said on Fox television,[6]

> You may remember what they first told us back in February and March? They said we have to take radical steps in order to "flatten the curve.'" Well, 6 weeks later, we're happy to say that curve has been flattened, but it's likely not because of the lockdown. The virus just isn't nearly as deadly as we thought it was. . . . Hospitals never collapsed. Outside of a tiny number of places, they never even came close to collapsing

This fallacy of "Any measures implemented soon enough to work will be seen as unnecessary" was the spoken version of the first Covid-19 predictive models that overestimated American death rates in the first months of the pandemic. The early models didn't take into account that people were going to change behavior—staying home, wearing masks, washing hands—and disease would slow down more than had been originally predicted by the model. This is one paradox of prevention: Interventions can achieve large overall health gains for whole populations but might offer only small advantages to each individual.[7]

During an infectious pandemic, prevention works by having people believe that prevention works. This is a second paradox of prevention. If a model inspires prevention, that model shapes the future it is predicting through the very act of prediction.

As Homer Simpson from the television show *The Simpsons* complained, "We're always buying Maggie vaccinations for diseases she doesn't even have."

* * *

CHAPTER 3

WE ARE NOT SURE WHO PUBLIC HEALTH IS FOR

W ho is public health for exactly? Who is this public, this Us anyway? In our trouble with these questions lays the third explanation for our undervaluing the public health perspective.

Public is an odd, shape-shifting word. It is a noun—The Public— and also an adjective—Public health. As an adjective, public implies something not concealed, open to general observation, sight, or cognizance. More, it suggests *easily* seen, prominent, conspicuous even (i.e., the opposite of private). It has a related meaning when used to modify authority. A public authority has an official or pro- fessional position of general influence or authority. Health care is concerned with an individual's private health, whereas public (ac- cording to the *Oxford English Dictionary*) health is "not restricted to the private use of any person or persons." To be public spirited is to be devoted to or directed to the promotion of the general welfare, no limits applied. But the word "public" allows an odd blurriness in usage and meaning.

As a noun, the public reads as singular but denotes plural, in the same way that community and nation evoke the plural (although these latter terms have boundaries—a person can be outside the community or not part of a nation). But in the term "public

Me vs. Us. Michael D. Stein, Oxford University Press. © Oxford University Press 2022.
DOI: 10.1093/oso/9780197637562.003.0004

health," the Public seems limitless because it is an abstraction. The "public" doesn't exist like a carpenter or a jazz singer does; it does not define itself through individuals.

Academics interested in public health and in words, and perhaps disappointed in how abstract and philosophical the notion of "the public" is, now sometimes refer to "population" health rather than "public" health. The term *population* encapsulates; it suggests a group with limits. An individual is clearly in the population or outside it. A population is countable (though dynamic—people move away, people die), and this is important in that countable people, by means of vote or protest, can have a say over the decisions that affect their lives. Populations share characteristics, such as where people live—a town, state, country—or in other instances, kinship, a health insurance plan, or a condition such as pregnancy or high blood pressure. Population sounds more scientific than public. And unlike public health, population health also has no connotation of government (the public sector) or politics.

Still, "public" has a warmer and more expansive and embracing feel than "population" and so remains above the door jambs of educational institutions. More important, because of its hybrid nature, its adjective–noun duality, public health suggests not only a perspective but also a set of functions in the world. Public health practice is a set of efforts that include disease surveillance and prevention (Ebola and water quality monitoring), policy-setting, community planning, and implementation for a specific population (e.g., getting air conditioning to the elderly in a heat wave) or a wider group.

Maybe it's this: Public health practice is not about the absence of the individual but, rather, the presence of a multitude-listening awareness, an attunement of the mind's ear and orientation of the spirit toward a group. It is the positive counterpoint to what the individual wants, and to individual autonomy.

* * *

In the summer of 1963, a deadly and highly contagious smallpox outbreak swept through the capital of Sweden. An American tourist, having spent 4 days in Sweden, headed home, feeling well and with no signs of illness. When she arrived in New York and couldn't prove she had been vaccinated against smallpox, health officials ordered her quarantined in a government hospital.

Her daughter, a lawyer, brought a federal lawsuit, requesting her release. There was no evidence that this traveler was exposed to smallpox, she had no symptoms, and, her daughter argued, the Swedish outbreak was on the decline weeks before her mother arrived in Stockholm. Here, the risk to the public comes face-to-face with an individual's rights. If you were the judge, how would you decide?

Quarantine orders require exposure or *potential* exposure to a contagious disease. This traveler might present some tiny, but ultimately incalculable, risk of carrying smallpox. If our traveler, in fact, wasn't actually exposed but was nonetheless held against her will, only she suffered. If she were released, there would be a small indeterminable risk of an outbreak. Your judgment on the case is likely to have less to do with evidence of actual exposure or infection than with making a safe decision for *the public*. In this instance, I would guess you have less sympathy for the individual and more concern for the community.

The judge in the actual case rejected the daughter's petition and ordered the mother involuntarily held for 2 weeks.[1] Judges are wary of releasing individuals who might have a communicable disease, and wary of contradicting the judgment of health officials. Neither judges nor health officials want to make a mistake that could be tragic. In this context, judges and health officials choose Us over Me (when the me can be contagious).

As a society, we demand that our health officials and judges be cautious about holding any one of us against our will. In order to involuntarily confine an individual, both the characteristics of the disease and the characteristics of the individual must be taken into account. How contagious is the infection? If you are unlucky enough to be exposed to this individual, what is the probability you will get sick or die? How long is an infectious person infectious, and do symptoms mark the beginning or end of infectiousness? (Each of these questions that guide the study of public health, by the way, is answered only by studying many people with such an infection.) Are there steps other than quarantine that might suffice to limit public risk? There is a wide spectrum of actions, such as daily monitoring, that infringe to a lesser extent on individual liberty than quarantine. The degree of intrusion into individual liberty should match the degree of risk to the public. These are policy and law questions, but also public health questions. The judge in the smallpox case was doing public health work. The judge chose Us.

When scientifically supported and necessary, quarantine helps garner trust among the public that it will be protected from real risks and not subjected to arbitrary coercion. Such trust, in turn, can encourage public cooperation with more general public health recommendations to prevent the spread of disease. In the best case, quarantine orders help protect the individual and the community. In the worst case, the quarantine regulations fail to adequately respect individual rights.

* * *

Public health has historically been a series of fitful, episodic responses to local threats.

In the 1790s, yellow fever (a disease we don't see in the United States anymore) was an East Coast epidemic responded to by quarantining ships, isolating individuals, fumigating houses, cleaning streets, removing garbage, and draining swamps. This set of measures, organized by temporary municipal "boards of health" with police powers, became public health.

Nearly 60 years after the woman flew home from Sweden, the cruise ship *Diamond Princess* carried, across miles of open sea, Covid-19 and the freight of the Me vs. Us problem.[2]

The *Diamond Princess* was headed toward port in Yokohama, Japan, in early February 2020 when the captain announced on the intercom that a passenger on the ship had tested positive for coronavirus 9 days earlier. Coronavirus was newly discovered, lethal for a significant number of persons infected, and had no treatment. With no available therapies, prevention of infection was the necessary means of saving lives. The captain had delayed sharing this unfortunate information until the final night of the 2-week voyage, February 3, after the last evening on-board parties and shows. He told all passengers to stay in their rooms until further notice. They would have to remain on ship an extra day to get screened to learn who had been exposed.

Medical officers on the ship started going door to door, taking temperatures, asking about coughs. Those who were older, symptomatic, or who had contact with the original patient were tested first. Yet guests came out the next morning and lined up at buffet tables for meals, sat together, and shared salt shakers and restrooms. This was the first in a series of subpar infection containment measures.

On February 5, the captain announced there were 10 infected persons on board. Nonetheless, crew members still shared rooms and sick crew members still worked above deck. Medical staff worked without full protective gear, gloves, or masks. As did the hundreds of health officials who came aboard to help with paperwork, testing, and screenings. New cases were announced daily, but sometimes the passengers only learned fellow passengers were infected via social media as the health ministry hundreds of miles away confirmed test results. Passengers counted the ambulances that pulled up at the dock to cart away the infected. On the fifth day, face masks were finally provided. Hallways were patrolled to prevent persons from sneaking out for a walk to get some air. Air, the medium of public health, was not to be shared. An extra day on the ship became a 2-week quarantine.

Nineteen percent of the 3,711 passengers and crew were infected.[3] With hundreds of infections and two deaths, the cruise ship became its own category in the initial World Health Organization indexing of coronavirus. Before the 2 weeks of quarantine were up, Americans were evacuated, the infected and uninfected together, separated in their getaway plane by a plastic curtain. After 14 days, the remaining passengers were released without having taken a valid Covid-19 test and remixed into the general Japanese population. At least one was later found to be infected, and perhaps had spread the infection.

We recognize the effect of our neighbors' health on ours during an infectious outbreak managed imperfectly. But do we imagine that we can ever manage an outbreak perfectly? Even our neighbors who look well, who "test negative," can be a threat.

Six weeks after the *Diamond Princess* event, the United States was shut down. Do such large-scale quarantines work? Do they save lives? Can they change the course of a rapidly escalating epidemic? These are new empirical questions.

During Covid-19, we were asked to value Us over Me. But the Me rule was deeply engrained. Ask anyone who rushed to a brunch or a bar as soon as they could. Ask anyone who refused to wear a mask.

* * *

For each individual, it's reasonable to measure health along a continuum, as I mentioned previously. When a person is recovering from Covid-19, she is healthier today than she was yesterday (healthier in the many senses; she's breathing better, she has more energy, it's easier for her to walk around and do what she wants to do). Let's apply this continuum-of-health idea to a population and stick with the example of obesity. We can probably agree that severe obesity is an indicator of poor health in that it puts a person at greater risk for diabetes, vascular disease, and several types of cancer and often limits that individual's daily activities and ability to function normally, our wider definition of health.

Take New York City as a case study—some New Yorkers are underweight and some are a little overweight and some are obese. We'd probably agree that if 40% of the residents of Manhattan are obese versus 30% of Staten Islanders, we'd say Staten Islanders were healthier (assuming all other underlying conditions are equal across the boroughs); if the weight of the average male Staten Island resident was 175 pounds rather than the 185 pounds of the average Manhattanite, we would probably say the Staten Island citizens are healthier.

Healthier in this example refers to differences in the weight distribution of the population. Public (population) health is not about the presence or absence of health (or illness) in any one person; in this case, it is about how widespread and how frequently we see obesity in these two boroughs. This is different from Me thinking, which does not concern itself with who else is obese as long as I'm not. Us thinking has an interest in what the larger forces are that move obesity rates from 40% to 30% in New York City—those forces that affect New Yorkers individually but also change the composite health of those they live among. Us thinking forces us to consider causes of health (or obesity) in a different way.

The reason or reasons (causes) one person is obese—genes, an overconsumption of sugary foods, a foot injury that limits exercise—will not necessarily apply across the city. Do we think Manhattan residents are, on average, heavier because they have worse genes, more intransigent appetites, or more heel spurs than Staten Islanders? The distribution of obesity *across* boroughs may have different causes than the causes of individual differences *within* the population of each borough.

Let's presume further that the prices of sugary drinks and vegetables are similar across boroughs. Let's say there is something in the environment of Staten Island that results in lower average weights—I'm making this up—more sunshine each day due to fewer skyscrapers which somehow melts away weight. Wouldn't we want to know about this unexpected factor? If we wanted to shift the population weight curve toward healthier, we could try to address the sunshine deficit (take down some buildings) in the Manhattan natives, thereby improving the health of the entire population in one fell swoop, rather than one person at a time.

We surely want to know what causes obesity in ourselves and our family and friends. But it's just as important to understand about the broader ways in which we can prevent obesity and shift the average weight curve of the population. We want to keep people and populations healthy. Public health practitioners are always asking about conditions and context: Is there something in the environment?

What if we learn that the "environmental" cause of obesity is not a lack of sunshine growing up but, rather, a lack of money (which leads to people eating more of the cheapest possible, most calorie-dense and processed food, for instance)? It would be difficult enough to get the Manhattanites to knock down some big buildings. But now do we have to solve poverty in Manhattan to reduce obesity?

* * *

Forty years ago, America's health—that is, the life expectancy of its population—was in the top half of all the high-income countries.[4] Today it's at the very bottom. Life expectancy here is lower than in countries such as Chile and Costa Rica. What happened?

From 1950 to 1980, the United States experienced a high economic growth rate and the lowest level of inequality in human history. Then growth stalled. Tax rates on corporations and wealthier individuals declined. The life expectancy of the richest quintile of 50-year-old Americans increased, as one might expect. Less well recognized, however, is that the life expectancy of the middle 60% of Americans did not budge much at all, and the life expectancy of the poorest 20% of Americans decreased. The trends for men and women were similar.

Income inequality—such as the share of income captured by the top 10% of Americans—increased during these 30 years. At the same time, our investment in health care skyrocketed compared to that of other countries. For those who could afford them, the prices we paid for medications and procedures reflected the value we placed on self-improvement. Yet average life expectancy of Americans began to decline compared to that of other countries with less inequality, less poverty.

Do factors beyond wealth[5]—such as where one lives and race and gender, some of the lines creating the hula hoop's hair in Chapter 2—affect longevity? To answer, let me use a slightly different measure of life expectancy—the likelihood that at birth you will live until age 70 years. This probability can be measured county by county across the United States where census data are collected. It can give us an insight into whether regional differences, or gender or race, matter for health.

Let's start with place.[6] White males born in the 10% most healthy counties have a 77% probability of survival to age 70 years, but only a 61% chance if born in the 10% least healthy counties. This disparity begs the question: What is it about a place that makes it healthier? Something about the attitudes of city living versus small town life? Or is it Northern versus Southern culture? More likely, it's something about the people who live there.

Gender and race matter. Females have a 13% better chance of reaching age 70 years than men. Whites have better chances of survival than Blacks—on average a whopping 17 percentage points higher for men and 12 for women. Putting these statistics together, we come up with one of the most stunning and disconcerting public health conclusions: 82% of White females can expect to live until age 70 years, whereas only 54% of Black males may have that expectation.

Geographic mortality inequities—less likely to survive to age 70 years in cities and in the South—are not inherent in location. Hidden within place are often racial differences, and within racial differences there are variations in other characteristics. Most of the Black–White gap in health is related to differences in education (more is healthier), in part due to how it plays out in occupation, income, and marital status (married is healthier). But these differences are more notably due to the dramatic effects of racial segregation on schooling, employment, and single parenthood.[7] Poverty is related to many other drivers of health—housing, transportation, incarceration, and food choice, for instance. But race and racism and poverty are terribly, inextricably bound in the United States, regardless of place and gender, because race, made-up system that it is, carries with it the experience of racism, which contributes to elevated health risks, from beginning to end, from preterm birth to premature death.

Of course, for an individual, we can't ever say that less education, or being single, or being a male caused that person to die before age 70 years or live to 100 years. There is a long list of possible contributing factors that could be included in a Me perspective on life expectancy—psychological stress, family history, smoking, sedentariness, self-control, job insecurity, and on and on. Life expectancy research does not permit evaluation of the specific health behaviors of those who died, or even of the health care they received. A public health perspective on premature death, because it focuses on an entire population, can only weigh a notably shorter list of contributors, ones that can be collected for analysis from nearly all of us, such as at the time of a census, like gender, race, and poverty. Each of us lives with a combination of genetic, biologic, and sociologic factors that matter; some of these are fixed (genes, birth sex, race), but others (poverty, social mobility) can be influenced by the context and conditions of our lives.

* * *

What if you don't believe that wealthy Europeans outlive wealthy Americans? What if you're *not* poor or *don't* feel the need to examine inequality? The public health voice sounds to you like a fable: "Once upon a time there was a country where 40% of people of one color were in prison . . .," "Once upon a time 82% of one group of people could expect to live until 70 whereas only 54% of another group may have that expectation . . .," "Once upon a time there was a country without universal health care . . .," "Once upon a time . . .".

Think of how much work one has to do to convince the listener of the reality of poverty, particularly when the listener's friends and children and partner are not experiencing it. The listener will have so many questions: Once upon a when exactly? Where? Who were these people? On what authority do you tell me about this? Why are you telling me, what do you want me to do?

Even the sympathetic listener doesn't know what to do with such public health tales, and feels badly she doesn't.

Now compare these abstractions to "My uncle was in a car accident and lost an eye," "My brother fell off a ladder and broke his femur," or "My needle biopsy was positive for cancer." The reality effect is strong and immediate. Why am I telling you? Because it happened to me and people I know. This reality effect is a powerful tool. You have the listener listening and feeling and the whole battle to help—to make them believe and to care—seems possible. All questions dissolve.

On the other hand, Public Health feels like its *insisting* on truth.

We live in a moment when all listeners and readers have tired of "Once upon a time there was a country . . ." and can now only accept accounts that speak directly to themselves. Once upon a time feels too inexact, too distant, appears to require too much effort, is too difficult to believe. People living in a 24-hour news culture have enough real medical stories to occupy them without being bothering with fairy tale lands of misery and imagined disadvantaged folks.

And so we have the third reason that public health gets underestimated.

* * *

CHAPTER 4

THERE IS LITTLE PRIVATE MONEY TO BE MADE IN PUBLIC HEALTH

If we're not sure whom public health serves—because it's invisible, because we're not thinking about water quality or food inspection or disease tracking on most days—we're certain about who consumes medical services. Consumption—money spent—has to take center stage in any discussion of health in America.

At first look, obesity would appear to be the classic Me condition. Despite our current nod to body positivity, the weight loss industry entices more than 100 million dieters into paid programs each year. Dieters typically makes four or five attempts per year in a $72 billion industry. There is money to be made in Me care. There are 5 million diet books sold each year, about half of all books in the health and fitness category. Each year brings a newly popular approach—keto, cave, wheat, zone, 20/20, intermittent fasting—each with the same promise: This is the one. The one with the best and singular plan, the new secret, the easy-to-follow steps, all painless. A celebrity endorsement helps. Medically supervised meal replacements, phone app–directed commercial diets, sold one by

Me vs. Us. Michael D. Stein, Oxford University Press. © Oxford University Press 2022.
DOI: 10.1093/oso/9780197637562.003.0005

one, which the dieter will need for years. Of course, no doctor has ever provided the solution to weight loss. If she had, there would only be one book, one slimming attempt that ended in success.

Being overweight, in our common understanding, is always an individual "problem," a Me problem. As a physician, I was trained to think of obesity as a behavioral issue: the person who drinks supersized soda rather than water, the person who watches 8 hours of television rather than taking walks. There is a cascade of personal choices that leads to obesity. Therefore, there must be a hundred different "personalized" ways to lose weight. Pick one. Buy one.

Diet books and videos and programs, weight loss pills and surgeries (all seemingly simple and certain), are moneymakers. These products offer treatments. They are marketed and sold to individuals. There are industries and entrepreneurs looking to get rich from millions of purchases by millions of people. This is not an indictment of money-making; it is an indictment of outcomes. Addressing obesity through a medical Me approach hasn't worked. Today, 42% of the population is obese.[1]

* * *

Health care, beyond the diet industry, is driven by money, perhaps to our detriment. Nearly half of Americans report having delayed or skipped medical care because of the cost. When you put off care, your cancer grows and it's harder to treat, more expensive to treat; outcomes are worse too. If you receive chemotherapy or immunotherapy, oncologists now use the term "financial toxicity" to talk about the cost of the drugs; high costs produce side effects, such as bankruptcy or less use of appropriate treatment, skipping doses to save money.

The price of insulin, on the list of miracle drugs, is 10 times higher in the United States than in Canada. If you ration your insulin until your next paycheck, you may die of diabetes. Americans who can afford the trip travel to Canada buy insulin there. On the other hand, it's unreasonable to travel to Canada for a magnetic resonance imaging scan because the country has one-fourth the number of machines as the United Sates does and there may be a wait list. The same discrepancy applies if you need a heart operation; Canada has one-third the number of surgeons. Americans get nearly unlimited numbers of scans and surgeries (if we have the insurance or cash), yet Canadian cancer and heart attack survival is as good as that in the United States. We overprovide high-priced services; we pay our providers about double what their Canadian counterparts earn. In some ways, spending too much money harms us by inducing us to believe in quantity as a substitute for quality. We overuse tests, like computed tomography scans, that deliver unnecessary radiation. We overuse pain treatment and end up with an opioid overdose epidemic that hasn't happened to our north.

I don't mean to compare the United States only to Canada. When we compare us to ourselves, we see that those living in geographic regions where we spend more money for health care are not the ones with the better health outcome.[2] Money spent on health care does not guarantee longer life.

Eighteen percent of the U.S. gross domestic product pays for health care (it was 5% in 1960). Yet 10% of the population is uninsured; if health care were less expensive, we'd probably find a way to pay for their care. Warren Buffett calls medical costs "the tapeworm of American economic competitiveness" (Berkshire Hathaway annual shareholder meeting, 2017, https://www.

yahoo.com/news/buffett-medical-costs-tapeworm-american-economic-competitiveness-220647855.html, Accessed 3/26/22). Auto companies claim that paying health benefits for workers raises the cost of each car by $1,500. Conversely, the cost of employer-covered health insurance for an employee with a family of four is the cost of buying a Toyota Corolla every year. Health insurance costs account for 60% of the cost of hiring a low-wage worker.

What we get from all this spending is *speed*. We are impatient, and there is no place in the world where you can get a knee replacement or a visit with a medical specialist faster. But in the broadest terms, we are spending more and getting less health, even if this all happens quickly.

The United States has among the lowest national life expectancies in the high-income world. Some people think this is a health care problem. It is, but only indirectly. The cost of medical care sucks governmental spending away from schools, from environmental and housing programs, from children's nutritional programs, from addressing the conditions and contexts of our lives. Lowering the cost of medical care won't improve life expectancy because there's little evidence that health care augments it. But changing to a public health perspective might.

* * *

Before Covid-19 arrived, we had lost interest in public health. Perhaps in part this disinterest came about because it seemed that the great victories of public health happened long ago. In the first half of the 20th century, public health interventions focusing on water and sanitation, and some decline in poverty, led to nearly all of the increase in life expectancy in the United States in that era. The amazing rush of vaccines midcentury—polio, measles, rubella, mumps—had conquered formerly common killers, such that later vaccines for hepatitis A and B, for one type of pneumonia and one type of meningitis, seemed almost anticlimactic. Motor vehicle accident rates declined, but this improvement was offset partially as we drove more miles. In the second half of the century, public health interventions to cut smoking rates and control hypertension and lower cholesterol levels cut death rates of heart disease and stroke by two-thirds, but health care got the credit as we associated these improvements with new medications and more effective technology.

Our interest in public health planning also faded because we turned our attention to the growing costs of our medical system. Starting in the 1960s, dollars have flowed into health care at a rate that far outpaces inflation. Medicare and Medicaid expanded health insurance, opening the use of more services—from nursing homes to expensive prescription medications—which came to consume more than 20% of our federal budget.

The Affordable Care Act (ACA), signed into law in 2010, was an attempt to insure more Americans while lowering the growth rate of health care spending, but it also included provisions that indicated we should be taking public health seriously. The ACA established a public health fund worth $15 billion over 10 years—the Prevention and Public Health Fund—to reduce the leading causes of death and disability, and support early detection of and response to new health threats. But in the past decade, this fund has been repeatedly raided by both congressional parties to pay for other, sometimes non-health items. The fund was cut by more than $1 billion in 2018 alone to help cover the costs of a bipartisan budget bill.

That same year, 2 years before coronavirus popped up, the Centers for Disease Control and Prevention (CDC) was forced to slash its efforts to prevent global disease outbreak by 80% because funding for the program was running dry.[3] To save money, the CDC opted to focus on 10 priority countries and scale back in others, including China. Also cut was the Complex Crises Fund, a $30 million emergency response pool that was at the secretary of state's disposal to deploy disease experts in the event of a crisis. Many of the programs created to safeguard public health, including programs designed specifically to protect the country from pandemics, were reduced.

The effects of all of these cuts were felt in 2020. When the CDC announced plans to test people for Covid-19, only three of the country's 100 public health department laboratories—labs that had a long history of developing and disseminating tests for new microbes (and old ones)—were able to test for coronavirus immediately because budget cuts had reduced staffing.[4] Testing was delayed. Then the CDC failed technically; its first tests for Covid-19 were inaccurate. The CDC was ill-prepared for a pandemic, its staff gutted, its systems rusty, muzzled by toxic politics.

As the nation's local and state public health officials confronted a pandemic, many of them made their situation clear: They were heading into a crisis without the resources they needed. In the decade before the diminishment of the CDC's global disease outbreak budget, local and state health departments had lost nearly a quarter of their workforce, 50,000 jobs nationwide, according to the National Association of County and City Health Officials. Most departments were short-staffed, overworked, and underfunded chronically when the initial supplemental congressional coronavirus funding was approved. Only 1/10th of the new congressional monies went to state and local health departments, which were eager to hire epidemiologists and increase laboratory capacity.

The creation of a healthy country takes sustained effort over many years, supported by collective investment and the best science. A panel studying the public health system in the United States, in the years before Covid-19, found that the country would need an additional $4.5 billion annual investment to protect national security and "create the conditions in which people can be as healthy as possible."[5]

"The conditions"; my colleague Lucas' language of "shared social and economic context." Conditions and context. Shared. By definition these are not Me concerns. They are the Us concerns of public health.

Public health's share of total health expenditures in the United States reached a high of 3.2% in 2002, before again declining recently. Ironically, in 1932, the report "Medical Care for the American People," written by the President of the American Public Health Association, recommended the reorganization of medical practice while lamenting the woeful state of public health. At the time of the report, only 3.3 cents of the "medical dollar" was spent on public health.[6] Slightly higher than today (2.6%), in the days of a pandemic.

* * *

The history of public health is sometimes confused with the history of contagions or outbreaks. It's not difficult to understand why. Forever, most sudden threats to populations were infectious: scarlet fever, typhoid fever, smallpox. We are still focused on infectious disease: Covid-19. These days most federal public health dollars flow from the CDC (and also from the U.S. Food and Drug

Administration) for functions such as epidemiological surveillance, immunization services, disease prevention programs, and the operation of public health laboratories: a suite of epidemic intelligence services.

What doesn't get counted in most current tallies of public health spending? Sewage treatment, water supplies protection, pollution abatement. We expect these services; they are part of public health's invisibility, and also its history.

From the beginning, public health measures were aimed at filth and garbage, thought to be the miasmic causes of poor health. Once upon a time, and still (in certain places), human waste appeared on the street, running water was rare, sewers rarer. Before the term "public health" came "public hygiene." Sanitary science was the rage in the 1800s, and business leaders recognized that an unhealthy environment hindered community growth; sanitary reform was wealth-creating. Public hygiene hadn't split apart from medicine yet; doctors constituted the earliest Boards of Health in Boston, Baltimore, Philadelphia, and Washington, DC.

By taking an interest in the tens of millions of new immigrants who arrived at the beginning of the 20th century, and the effects of poverty—disease-spreading schools, hazardous workplaces, dilapidated tenements, the growing infant mortality rates—public health authorities went too far for many doctors. Soon public health was attacked as socialistic and bureaucratic by the growing sector of private practice physicians. Soon public health "was relegated to a secondary status, less prestigious than clinical medicine, less amply financed, and blocked from assuming the higher-level functions of coordination and direction."[7]

* * *

The division between the Me and Us perspectives drives federal funding priorities, channels our resources ($11,000 spent per person per year for health care vs. $286 per person for public health, which is another way of saying public health is 1/40th as important as medicine), distorts our media coverage of health, and affects our conversations.[8,9] The dominance of the Me is dangerous, as we've begun to see, leaving us less healthy, less long-lived as a nation than we might be.

We value health dearly. What we value, however, as evidenced perhaps best by our expressed spending preference, is the attainment of individual health—preferably at a rapid pace—my capacity to be as healthy as I can be, and to spend as much money as I want to optimize my health. This is, of course, consistent with an American adherence to the notion of individual capacity for limitless achievement above all else.

Discussions of health care versus public health seem to be zero sum, and there are only so many conversations about health in a world that also concerns itself with entertainment, politics, shopping, weddings, sports, gossip, war. Every health care conversation about Medicare-for-all or private insurance coverage, the newest robotic surgery or genetic test, and the latest report from the precision medicine front takes the place of a public health conversation about liquor store density, soda and cigarette taxes, or vaccination rates, all of which more broadly influence life expectancies. Those issues that we think about and talk about, we act on. How we divide our thinking between medical and public health perspectives matters.

* * *

The Master Settlement Agreement of 1998 (MSA) between the attorneys general of 46 states and the four largest cigarette manufacturers in the United States ended the largest civil litigation settlement in history. Four years earlier, a number of states sued the manufacturers under state consumer protection and antitrust laws, asserting that the industry's deceptive and misleading conduct constituted a wrong against the public and that cigarettes contributed to health problems that led to significant costs to state health care systems. The states alleged that they were being forced to pay smoking-related health care costs that should properly be the responsibility of the cigarette companies, which had lied to the public about the addictiveness of nicotine, marketed to children, and suppressed information about the dangers of smoking.

The MSA imposed restrictions on the sale and marketing of cigarettes by participating cigarette manufacturers. In addition, the tobacco industry was required to pay the settling states billions of dollars annually, in perpetuity, because health care costs due to their citizens' smoking-related illnesses will likely continue indefinitely.

The MSA stated that its primary purpose was to decrease youth smoking and promote public health in the respective states. But it did not contain any provisions requiring states to allocate settlement revenues to tobacco prevention and smoking cessation. State legislatures were responsible for deciding how the money was spent.

As of July 2018, the participating manufacturers had paid over $126 billion to the settling states, and less than 1% of these funds were earmarked for state tobacco prevention programs for children or for helping smokers quit. In 2017, 17 states did not allocate *any* of their MSA payments to tobacco prevention and cessation programs.[10]

Although the majority of these funds were used by legislators to pay for budget shortfalls (including paying Medicaid expenses or tax credits), a significant portion was diverted for new health care projects such as building new cancer centers, the funding of medical schools, and for biomedical research. The adequate funding of public health and prevention was ignored; medical care provided much more immediate and tangible results, and political payoff.

* * *

Despite the increase in diet books and a growing list of new programs and dollars spent, obesity has increased dramatically in the past 50 years. Why is it that only a tiny percentage of people who try to lose weight on a diet succeed? Why is it that many people actually gain more weight than they lost following their diet?

The answer is that obesity is relational; people don't get heavy or thinner alone; most times, someone—often someone who shares a refrigerator with the person attempting to lose weight— is watching along the way. Which suggests that excess weight is not merely a Me problem. Obesity is certainly biologically driven, but it is also social. What can another person do to help? Two people are a group, the smallest group from a public health perspective, but a group nonetheless. If that other person can cajole, cheerlead, limit, reward, deter, they serve as a source of accountability. Sometimes there is only one other person who influences the dieter's decisions; sometimes there are others around the table. Sometimes what first appears to be a relational influence is actually more surrounding, a cultural influence ("This is how we eat in the South" or "This is how Latino families cook"). Context matters too. We eat at home and on the way home, at work and after work, at school in cafeterias and from backpacks. What food is available in the stores and schools of our neighborhood, and what's affordable?

This leads to a practical question: What broader public health policies can multiply or undermine the effect of a "personalized" weight loss plan?

We consume 23% more calories, on average, than we did 50 years ago. These excess calories are a function of the type and quantity of food we consume. There is not only food (and its calories) but also food systems that dictate the production, processing, distribution, preparation, and, finally, the consumption of food. Food systems have changed in these 50 years; there is increased processing and expanded food diffusion, such that convenient, energy-dense foods (sugar-sweetened drinks, candy, cakes) have become more available. These are heavily promoted to appeal to consumers, and their prices have fallen in comparison to those of less energy-dense foods such as fruits and vegetables. This price discrepancy has contributed to caloric overconsumption, worsened by larger portion sizes. In other words, the individual trying to diet is fighting food systems and buying and eating contexts, which are shaped by social and cultural influences, scientific advances, policies and regulations (corn and sugar subsidies), and economic factors. These influences affect all of us, the dieters and non-dieters alike.

Which food system features are most strongly related to caloric overconsumption and obesity? If we wanted to do a feasible, effective intervention to reach a healthier average weight for a whole society, what would we do? It's unlikely there is a single answer, and we don't know which interventions might act synergistically.

At the same time, despite high rates of obesity, the rates of hunger throughout the country are also substantial, paradoxically.

Because obesity is about food consumption, food policies matter. Yes, the individual puts the food into their mouth, but what food and how much are shaped by family, community, and societal decisions and by local programs as much as by federal and state taxes affecting farmers, truckers, grocers, and eaters. Eliminating corn subsidies or taxing sugary drinks, figuring out ways to decrease the price of vegetables—policies drawn from a public health perspective—represent a different approach to thinking about weight loss. The public health approach to obesity is *preventive*. The health goal is to prevent obesity, to address its root causes rather than step in with medications and bariatric surgery when nearly half the population is obese. We don't really know if dramatic changes to taxes or subsidies could produce the desired preventive result of fewer overweight people because we've never tried them at scale for an extended period. We haven't done so because such policies are not "business friendly." Prevention policies deprive large corporations of profits. On the other hand, we know that the *treatment* of obesity is a moneymaker (Weight Watchers reported $1.4 billion in revenue in 2020) because for some people, over the short term, treatment seems to work and we're willing to pay for results, repeatedly, endlessly.

There is money to be saved (which, unfortunately, is not thought of as the opposite of money *to be made*, and it's always a matter of who is making or saving money) if large-scale preventive policies work. If people who lived in Manhattan say, on average, weighed less there would be less diabetes, fewer cardiovascular events and hospitalizations, and fewer cancers in Manhattan, which in turn might lower how much Manhattanites spend on health services, which in turn could lower health insurance premiums that pay for overpriced medical care. Still, if one goal of food policy to reduce obesity is to save federal or state monies, the primary goal is to improve health.

* * *

We value what we pay for. What product does public health "sell"? Who is the public health consumer? What business is public health in, and why does public health have no brand recognition? If public health workers are city, state, and federal employees, chances are there's not a lot of money floating around. Making policy is not about making money or branding. I've never met a rich public health practitioner.

But as someone who wants people (including me) to live longer, I get frustrated sometimes that at the core of the American point of view is the belief that private enterprise is intrinsically more important than public enterprise.

* * *

Policymakers are always asking about return on investment (ROI). The ROI is the benefit minus the cost expressed as a proportion of the cost of a policy; for any intervention, we can derive an ROI. Does prevention, the deterrence work of public health, have a good ROI?

Researchers have calculated the ROI for four types of public health interventions performed at either the local or the national level: health protection, health promotion, legislative interventions, and those related to health care delivery.[11] Health protection interventions, such as vaccinations, have a median ROI of 34, which means that half of the interventions save at least

$34 for every $1 spent on them. (In the case of vaccinations, the savings comes from avoiding the cost of providing medical care for a case of measles or mumps). Not that every vaccine has a positive return. For example, in years for which the flu vaccine is a poor match for the actual influenza types that are infecting the public, the ROI can be as low as −21, meaning that it costs $21 to save $1 (not good). In years for which the vaccine matches the disease well, the ROI can be as high as 174, which again means every dollar invested yields a return of $174 plus the original investment back (investors sometimes use ROI and "rate of return" interchangeably). Such a high return occurs because disease and hospitalization and death are prevented—years of good health increase.

Health promotion interventions, including programs to prevent falls among older people or campaigns to get people to quit smoking, have a typical ROI of approximately 2. Returns can be higher if programs target high-risk people. Such targeting conserves resources without wasting them on people who are not likely to respond or be in need of help—for example, targeting flu vaccines to the elderly rather than to young, healthy workers. Improvements in the built environment, such as laying new sidewalks to encourage walking, and traffic safety programs, have a typical ROI of approximately 5. Childhood programs are particularly potent (we'll return to this later); lead paint removal saves $221 for every $1 spent.

Legislative interventions, such as ones addressing obesity, can make major differences, with a median rate of return of 47. They are relatively cheap and can target behavior at a national level. For instance, a tax on sugar-sweetened beverages has an estimated rate of return of 55.

Health care interventions—new medication for macular degeneration or a new chemotherapy agent for stomach cancer—have an ROI, on average, of 3.2, which is notably lower than those of local public health interventions at 4.1 or upstream legislative ones, averaging 46. But no one likes to cut spending on health care or health care interventions.

The median ROI for public health programs has been approximately 14.3. A business person would not believe the pitch for any investment that provided a 1,430% return; it would sound too good to be true, and an investor would ask which studies of programs never got written up in such a summary because they *didn't* do so well. Yet that's the data, providing a strong case for public health spending.

With a 1,430% return, why is public health considered a soft target for budget cuts by legislators? Because the benefits of public health interventions—unlike personal health care interventions—tend to accrue over the long term, long after politicians and policymakers have moved on. Because though large and certain at the population level, benefits are seen as small and uncertain for any particular individual (i.e., they are not Me-focused). Because public health interventions are often opposed by powerful commercial interests (e.g., corn syrup manufacturers and soda makers), and our political representatives are financially disinclined toward Us interventions.

But public health interventions are tricky in another sense. "Savings" imply a future. If a public health program is not instituted (or cut by legislators), the ailments and deaths that might be avoided would be occurring in a time yet to come. They must be imagined. Teen pregnancies, suicides, and disease outbreaks are concerning, but if and when they arrive, they can be blamed on other things rather than the underinvestment in prevention.

* * *

Any prevention intervention has start-up costs. Let's say we want to turn our public health attention to how to decrease recidivism among incarcerated persons, a population notable for its density of chronic medical conditions—substance use, mental health, hepatitis, hypertension—and for its poverty. Although generally young, prisoners are unhealthy. We know (from our previous ROI evaluation) that effective recidivism prevention programs exist and remaining out of jail is one way to improve health.

Government officials could write a contract that solicits a community organization to come up with a plan to keep people out of jail and could pay them federal or state funds to do the work. But what if the government outsourced the work in another way, ensuring that anti-recidivism services are still provided while the risk of financing such services is borne by private investors rather than the government? The investor who provides upfront financing for service delivery is only reimbursed by the government if predetermined outcomes are met. The contract could be written, for instance, such that an investor will receive a financial return of 2.5% if there is a 7.5% reduction in reoffending, when measured against a matched control group (to ensure any such reduction can be attributed to the investor's performance); higher reduction rates in reoffending would generate higher financial returns. A socially minded investor can foster promising preventative interventions while the actual service providers receive the necessary funds to scale-up existing work, and government purchasers only pay for successful programming. A win–win–win. Government saves on the cost of housing returned prisoners and passes on part of the savings to investors.

This partnering of a government office with private for-profit investors, social investors (who seek a blend of financial return and social good), or philanthropists to fund interventions that tackle difficult social problems is structured around a financial vehicle called a social impact bond (SIB).[12] (SIBs pay out financial returns only when specified social outcomes have been met, thus acting more like an equity product than a traditional bond which pays fixed interest for a set period.) SIBs have been around for a decade as a type of payment-by-results contract for public services provision. They were created as one answer to the eternal government question, How do we make use of scarce public resources in the most efficient way?

There will be scarce public resources after the Covid-19 crisis ends, when the depth of the federal deficit, generated to protect small businesses and the newly unemployed, sinks in and public spending for public health inevitably fades. As governmental spending goes down under the new austerity, this will almost certainly include decreases in public health spending.

In the post-Covid-19 United States, you'd think SIBs would then have even greater appeal to policymakers on both sides of the political aisle. They offer liberals an opportunity to expand service provision and conservatives a mechanism for private investment and involvement in public services delivery. If SIBs have the potential to foster innovation and to "scale up" evidence-based programs, the narrative would be that government-led public health efforts will take on the reflected glow of a new form of American business and profit-making, bringing market discipline to nonprofit service providers and improving the health of populations.

Why are there only about 10 SIBs in the United States? There would seem to be plenty of worthy ventures. Jail recidivism provides a promising target. It has a clearly measurable outcome—Did the person return to jail or not?—and a definable, finite population. But still, reducing recidivism is a massively complex problem (as most public health problems are), even if the outcome is simple. It requires liaising with (and perhaps changes in the practices of) several agencies involved in providing and supporting the target client group, including housing, medical benefits, and employment training; the impact is also inevitably shaped by the nature of the local employment market. It is possible that the investors' anti-recidivism campaign would be let down by failings in another part of the support system that former prisoners need if they are to have a reasonable prospect of improving their situation. SIBs do not guarantee simple mechanical fixes to problems that entail the reconfiguration of complex health and social conditions.

That there are so few SIBs suggests there are reservations on both sides, from government officials and from investors. From the government official's viewpoint, in situations in which government doesn't directly choose the actual services provider (as through a typical SIB contract), and the private investor picks poorly (trying to save money, they choose the lowest bidder) and the project fails, the government may still be blamed, doubly eroding trust in government accountability. After all, the jailed person and his family, friends, and neighbors would know only they were in a lousy program they assumed was paid for like any other. What if malpractice occurs by the investors' service provider? What if recidivism gets worse? The government would have no oversight and couldn't easily intercede.

In addition, some believe that SIBs are antithetical to public values, enabling the "financialization" of public services. Can commercial interests really be pursued for the public good? Isn't there a special risk of cutting corners for profit if they are focused mainly on marginalized groups such as prisoners? Do SIBs highlight the inherent conflict between the relative openness of public sector contracting and the closed nature of private financial arrangements? From the investor's standpoint, the question remains whether SIBs can generate meaningful financial returns. SIBs are technically difficult to commission and require complex contractual relationships between different actors, requiring long set-up times and steep transaction costs.

The Rikers Island anti-recidivism SIB in New York (tested rigorously in a randomized trial) was canceled after 3 years of operation, short of the 6 years it was contracted for, because it failed to meet its stated outcomes.[13] But could it still be viewed as a success? Private monies protected the government purchaser from investing in an intervention that did not deliver on its promises, but the intervention had a positive impact on some service recipients even though it did not meet its overall prespecified metrics. The creators of this anti-recidivist program argued that the benefits extended far beyond their health effects. Some participants reported improvement in literacy and job prospects. Persons helped by anti-recidivist programs not only produce costs savings to the criminal justice system but also, if employed, contribute tax dollars.

So far, there is limited evidence that SIBs produce better outcomes for service recipients or are more cost-effective than direct public financing for public services. If SIBs became widespread, maybe there would be private money to be made in public health. But doing public health for profit, from all the evidence at hand, SIBs included, is not easy.

A serious demerit for public health remains: There is little private money to be made in public health.

* * *

CHAPTER 5

PUBLIC HEALTH FRAMES ITS SUCCESSES INCORRECTLY

Social impact bonds typically take up prevention issues, promising savings for some outcome (a reincarceration, a traffic accident) in some imagined far-off time, which we like to believe may never happen to any member of a population (prisoners, drivers). Public health has a future-focused perspective. Because the outcome is far off, such public health interventions do not address an imminent threat that requires an immediate fix, the kind of outcome we often deem medical. Medicine has a present-focused perspective.

If you are exposed to a virus and knew there was a 1 in 1,000 chance that you had contracted a fatal disease, how much would you pay for the drug to cure it? Now turn the question around. How much would you need to be paid to be exposed to a 1 in 1,000 chance of getting the same fatal disease?

Economic theory says the two payments should be the same. Whatever you were willing to pay to rid yourself of a 1 in 1,000 chance of dying should be the same as what you needed to be paid to expose yourself to a 1 in 1,000 chance of dying. Yet people whose lives are only hypothetically on the line don't value the two equally. The answers are orders of magnitude apart.

Me vs. Us. Michael D. Stein, Oxford University Press. © Oxford University Press 2022.
DOI: 10.1093/oso/9780197637562.003.0006

People would pay $10,000 for the cure, but they would need to be paid $1 million to be exposed. That's paying 100 times more to avoid the chance of being infected with an incurable disease than for a cure for the same disease they had a 1 in 1,000 chance of catching. (Another public health question is: What would you pay *never* to be exposed to the pathogen?)

We seem to value prevention more than cure. So why, as a society, are we willing to pay for cure (the medical perspective) and not for prevention (the public health perspective)?

* * *

There are 350,000 house fires in the United States each year, causing 4,000 deaths. A functioning smoke alarm reduces this number by more than half, yet only half of all houses with fires have smoke alarms. Smoke alarms cost money and their distribution across communities requires supplies and personnel.

The Dallas Red Cross, Fire Rescue Department, and Injury Prevention Center worked together to hand out smoke detectors to 8,000 households in areas that were high risk due to high rates of previous fires, most often in low-income neighborhoods.[1] Over the next 5 years, residents receiving alarms observed 68% fewer fatal and nonfatal fire injuries compared with residents in houses in nearby neighborhoods who did not receive alarms. There was a strong return on investment, $3 for every dollar spent.

Public health is a smoke alarm. Covid-19 made clear that a disease anywhere is a disease everywhere. Fire spreads if not extinguished. Covid-19 demonstrated that public health consists of an alarm *before* and a response *after* the first case. Public health requires a surveillance and detection system and a battery (installed by workers) that sounds loudly when there's smoke. During the first days of Covid-19, public health was the smoke alarm alerting all that the health care system was about to burn.

It takes political will to spend money on a smoke detection system that might never be needed. The public health view is: You're not going to stop outbreaks from happening, but you can stop outbreaks from becoming epidemics. There are fires that spill over to unexpected places, but they don't have to burn down the world.

* * *

One of the most discussed triumphs of public health prevention in the 20th century was the reduction in motor vehicle fatalities. Although the number of drivers and vehicles increased by more than 10 times over the century, the annual death rate declined from 19 per 100 million vehicle miles traveled to 1.4, a 96% improvement.

In the 1930s, when cars were becoming popular, motor vehicle deaths increased markedly. There were two ways to deal with this problem. One was to say, "Cars don't kill, people kill." This suggests that the solution was to educate people about the risks of speeding and oblige them to prove their driving skills through regular road tests. The other solution was to admit that personal behavior matters but focus instead on the context, the conditions of operating a car, the basis of poor driving outcomes, as it were.

The improvement in motor vehicle-related fatalities has been attributed to the many changes set in motion in 1966 by the Highway Safety Act and the National Traffic and Motor Vehicle Safety Act, which authorized the federal government to set and regulate standards for motor vehicles and highways. American companies began to build cars with new safety features—headrests, energy-absorbing steering wheels, shatter-resistant windshields, safety belts, and, later, airbags and anti-lock brakes. Highways were redesigned, roads revamped with better delineation of curves (edge and center line stripes and reflectors), use of breakaway sign and utility poles, and improved illumination. Barriers were added, separating oncoming traffic lanes, and guardrails too. It is almost impossible to imagine a time without barriers, but this upgrade happened in my lifetime. Changes in driver and passenger behavior followed the enactment and enforcement of traffic safety laws that were reinforced by public education. There was new prosecution of laws against driving under the influence and underage drinking, and administration of safety belt, child safety seat, and motorcycle helmet use laws. Citizen- and community-based advocacy groups chipped in, taking critical roles against drinking and driving, in child-occupant protection, and in favor of graduated driver licenses for teenagers. It was a victory in prevention, it seemed, "driven" by public health policy.

But skeptics of prevention policy point to increases in traffic congestion, not this long list of creative regulations, as an equally sound explanation for the strong inverse association between decreased road fatality and miles traveled.[2] They suggest most of the increase in vehicle miles traveled occurs in and around large cities during rush hours. These are miles where mean and maximum traffic speeds approach standstill, and thus case fatality rates would have fallen without the institution of any public health measures. No one gets killed in a traffic jam. Much of the credit for the public health "achievement" then comes from the slow travel during peak hours of most vehicles.

* * *

Here's a classic public health experiment: The minister of transportation in the country of Fasternak recommends raising the speed limit from 56 to 64 mph for all vehicles, including trucks, on a specific highway connecting two medium-sized cities.[3] The stated justification is to gain the economic benefits of time saving from interurban travel at higher speeds. At the same time, she also recommends lowering the speed limit in highly crowded urban areas to 20 mph. It is predicted that even though there would be zero to two more deaths per year on the newly "high-speed" road, death tolls overall would drop by some eight to 10, as traffic would be diverted from higher risk (to pedestrians and cyclists) low-speed roads to high-speed roads.

The first month following the change to 64 mph is the worst ever for road death tolls on this highway. Sixty-one persons are killed, not one or two, with a marked rise in case fatality, an index of severity of crashes. There is a spillover rise in death toll on all other major highways and feeder roads.

Public health policies are exercises in human experimentation, in this case with the outcomes of death, injury, and disability. How is the decision to continue for 8 more months with the "experiment" after the first month's high death tolls allowed? The arguments include the fact that a raised speed limit does not *require* drivers to increase their speed. And other roads are available for those wishing a more leisurely drive. Objectors point out that in many prior studies raising speed limits on major roads has increased driving speeds and fatalities and that the minister's notable underestimate was predictable. Today, 30 years after this experiment was performed, the current estimate is that a 10% increase in travel speeds will produce a 43% rise in death rates.[4]

Transportation decisions weigh the economic benefits of fast transport of persons and goods against the costs of injury and death. Death and injury are considered an unwelcome but necessary price to be paid by an unlucky minority for increasing happiness, pleasure, and profit among the majority. It is a choice between the absolutist ethical principle that any preventable death is unacceptable, that life and its preservation are an ultimate value, and the principle of the greatest good for the greatest number of people.

The speed limit decision is not so different from the pathogen question of the previous section about what you would pay not to be exposed. How much death would you accept to live somewhere with (very modestly) higher speed limits? (No one would deny that people would hate 56 mph limits on high-speed roads.)

In some ways, this highway experiment also reflects the stark choice during the Covid-19 pandemic. How long do we remain in lockdown? For how long should we try to minimize individual risk, knowing that economic fallout will follow? When should normal human interaction proceed (with risk mitigated somewhat by masks and social distancing), knowing that deaths will rise with the return to pre-Covid-19 activity?

On roads, kinetic energy is the pathogen; the risk for injury is predicted by the combined effect of mass and speed. Heavier vehicles punish lighter ones; the probability of death among occupants of light vehicles colliding with heavy vehicles is extremely high. And higher speeds produce more deaths. The start of the 21st century has not reproduced the 20th century's reduction in motor vehicle fatalities because higher speed limits, raised in the 1990s, continue to this day. The death toll in the United States has remained in the range of 40,000 victims per year for two decades. We continue to observe that emptier roads and cities with fewer cars have higher case fatality rates, probably because people drive faster, supporting the speed = death equation. We sacrifice lives to the collective benefit of saving time and the thrill of acceleration.

Lower speed limit advocates note that the role of protecting the average driver may be similar to the public health role of protecting non-smokers from the risks of second-hand tobacco smoke. The risks for injury and death are increased not only for those who speed but also for those road users—passengers in high-speed cars, drivers of lower speed cars, and pedestrians–who are involuntarily exposed.

Often, public transport—trains and buses, modes of transportation with much lower risks—is unavailable, but there may be other remedies. In the United Kingdom, there has been a reduction by 40% in deaths in the past decade attributed to a network of speed cameras. These surveillance networks are sustainable because their revenues make them self-financing through speeding tickets. Why do we object to supervision? Is it the same reason that front seat belt use in the United States is lower than in most other high-income countries? Do we believe these personal "choices"— unharnessed speed—are expressions of liberty?

* * *

Here are two more point-of-view problems to consider.

Imagine that the United States is preparing for the outbreak of an unusual disease that is expected to kill 600 people. Two alternative programs to combat the disease have been proposed. Assume that the scientific estimate of the consequences of the programs are as follows:

If program A is adopted, 200 people will be saved.

If program B is adopted, there is a one-third probability that 600 people will be saved, and a two-thirds probability that no people will be saved.

Which of the two programs would you favor? Overwhelmingly, people choose A to save 200 lives with certainty.

How about the following:

If program C is adopted, 400 people will die.

If program D is adopted, there is a one-third probability that nobody will die and a two-thirds probability that 600 people will die.

Overwhelmingly, people choose D.

The two problems are identical. Except in the first case, when the choice is framed as a gain—lives saved—people elect to save 200 for sure (which mean 400 would dic for sure though the readers aren't thinking this way). In the second case, with the choice framed as a loss—people will die—most readers choose the opposite and the risk that everyone would die.

Your answers to the two problems should be identical—the way the problems differ should be irrelevant—but they aren't. This is pertinent to how we think about public health. Perspectives matter. What people want changes with the context in which the options are offered.

People do not choose between things. They choose between descriptions of things.

As in the fatal virus cure versus prevention scenario, public health workers should only talk about the number of people *saved*, not the number of cases *prevented*.

Another reason for our failing to appreciate public health is now apparent.

CHAPTER 6

PUBLIC HEALTH CAN ONLY INFREQUENTLY PERFORM RANDOMIZED TRIALS AND THEREFORE SEEMS LESS RIGOROUS

One in three Americans has prediabetes, a high blood sugar that is not high enough to qualify for the title of diabetic. Still, within 5 years, 70% of individuals with prediabetes will develop diabetes. Diabetes doubles the risk of having a stroke or heart attack and vastly increases one's chances of having kidney disease, experiencing nerve pain, or losing sight from retinal problems. Diabetes is the seventh leading cause of death and is the main reason why young women have heart attacks.

The vast majority of those with prediabetes are overweight, although not everyone who is overweight is prediabetic. If we could develop a comprehensive, relatively brief program that changes the trajectory from prediabetes to diabetes, we could save lives. The Diabetes Prevention Program (DPP) randomized approximately 3,200 prediabetic Americans to one of three interventions: a 16-week instruction in lifestyle change, a medication used to treat

Me vs. Us. Michael D. Stein, Oxford University Press. © Oxford University Press 2022.
DOI: 10.1093/oso/9780197637562.003.0007

diabetes that also showed evidence of preventing diabetes, or a placebo pill. The lifestyle intervention (changes in eating, increases in exercise) resulted in a 58% reduction in the incidence of developing diabetes 3 years later compared to the placebo pill, and it was twice as effective as the active medication in diabetes prevention. This effect lasted 10 years, well past the time of the clinical trial's end date.

The results of this diabetes prevention research were difficult to deny: Investigators had performed a *randomized clinical trial.* Those three magical words. Why do we consider randomized trial results the gold standard for proving an intervention works? By randomly assigning patients to one treatment or another, and by having participants stick to their assigned treatment during a period of strict observation, clinical trials rely on chance to create treatment groups with similar characteristics (gender, age). This random selection (think of how Powerball lotteries are drawn on television— numbered ping pong balls bouncing in a cage, one popping up after another to determine the winning sequence) does not allow the researchers any say in who joins a particular treatment group, and by doing so it precludes any human biases.

Randomization gives the best chance for a fair comparison of groups, minimizing one problem (baseline differences between groups) that might disrupt the chance of obtaining valid results; any differences in outcomes can be attributed to the intervention rather than preexisting differences between study participants in each group. The rigorous, controlled design and the statistical approaches that have evolved to evaluate randomized trials are codified and convincing. Clinical trials are reliable for determining the effectiveness of an intervention. Modern medicine has earned its reputation by performing randomized clinical trials; they monopolize our media attention.

But trials are laborious. They require meticulous standardization in measurements and process. They are sometimes slow and disrupt participants' lives during the trial period. Because they are expensive to perform, they often include only a small number of participants (which means chance may not, in fact, equalize groups) who are followed for too short a time. Therefore, randomized trials sometimes can't give a full picture of a treatment's safety if that treatment were to be applied over hundreds of thousands of people; a side effect that occurs in 1 in 1,000 people is unlikely to show up during a trial of only 100 people.

The randomized trial tells us what treatment works best, but no treatment works equally for everyone, and if we had even more granular patient data, perhaps we could manage high blood sugar better. Still, one could say there is not enough individualization in medicine today. We have tools now that can make use of our personal genetic profile and behaviors. We can sequence an individual's DNA somewhat inexpensively and bring it together with data acquired from sensors attached to the body—heart rate, temperature, sweat constituents—and perhaps this can enhance for a given individual the effective treatment identified by a trial. With patient care, it is one patient at a time, but now, with the help of genomics and modern technology, care can be even more efficient and more personal. More precise.

Yet as we seek greater medical precision, we recognize that not every health question can be answered through a randomized trial. We can't randomize one city to do contact tracing for Covid-19 patients and another to avoid this service. It is unacceptable to oblige some cigarette smokers but not others to pay a higher tax per pack. It is impossible to randomize some drivers to a road with a higher speed limit and other drivers to a road with a lower speed limit. To answer these public health questions, we need to do studies other than randomized trials.

* * *

Because not every health question can be answered through a randomized trial, rich and sophisticated research has evolved to examine the health effects of social policies or even memorable public events. Much of this research depends on natural experiments of such policies or events (something happens and there's a before and after that happening) that produce large (or small) cultural changes that find their way into the health of populations.

For instance, we know the expansion of Obamacare occurred in some states but not others. Can we compare health of the populations across those two types of states? Yes: Providing more low-income persons with Medicaid has led to decreased mortality overall (infant mortality in particular), and for certain specific groups (e.g., persons receiving dialysis for kidney failure), as well as reductions in rates of food insecurity, poverty, and home evictions, and improvements in measures of self-reported health and healthy behaviors such as diabetes management and quitting smoking in Obamacare expansion states.

Or what happens when an auto plant closes, an event that can shock a community or region? Researchers have found that persons living within the same labor market (commuting zone) of a plant closure go on to have increased rates of opioid overdose mortality compared to those living in other manufacturing regions without such closures.

Or what happens when race-based affirmative action programs for college admissions are banned in some states and not others?

Cigarette smoking and alcohol use increase among underrepresented minority 11th and 12th graders in those states with bans, suggesting banning affirmative action policies, devised as economic opportunity policies, may have important adverse spillover effects on health risk behaviors.

We can measure the self-reported mental health of African Americans before and after a highly publicized police shooting of an unarmed young Black person. Such measurements find detrimental effects following that death—effects not reported by White Americans after police shootings. A public event can harm the health of a particular community and of a nation.

These kinds of public health studies, analyses of specific events or policies, reveal discrete breaks in health behaviors and consequences timed with the trauma of a shock or the implementation of a new program. We will never be able to randomize such happenings or do "trials" of them. But such studies often reveal inequalities and provide better predictions about the future.

Randomized trials suggest that there is something a participant (and by extension anyone) can do to improve their health. They have a health care perspective: How can I fix what's wrong with me? These natural experiments of factories closing and citizens murdered suggest again that health across a population is contingent on contexts and conditions that are often out of an individual's control. They have a public health, a community-based perspective: What's wrong with us?

* * *

The DPP was a Me trial. It included the test of a potentially diabetes-preventing medication versus a behavioral approach to weight loss. Every individual enrolled received personal attention during their study involvement; the putative therapies focused on the individual. It had no Us component, strictly speaking, although the study investigators offered tricks to the behavioral group participants on how to interact with a world that triggered weight gain. The behavioral intervention included, for instance, how to read food labels, how to be aware of sugar content, and simple ways to be physically active. But the researchers did not attempt to change *the world* the prediabetic participants lived in. They did not plan a change in food policy, raising taxes on sugary beverages, or creating more green space so participants would have more enticing places to walk or bike.

Since the landmark DPP study, there have been massive efforts to get this behavioral program that showed such good effects in preventing diabetes into clinical practice and to extend its reach beyond its form as a Me recommendation. Why has it been vastly underutilized given its ability to drive down diabetes, a known killer, a major contributor to our lagging life expectancy?

The list of reasons is long. Doctors don't know about or have any idea how to "prescribe" behavior change programs. The program itself costs money to run, and the insurance reimbursement for such programs is inconsistent. Sixteen-week structured programs may be off-putting because of the effort required; a pill is likely more appealing. And after all, the participants in DPP did not *have* diabetes, a clinical label; they probably felt healthy in most instances; perhaps they didn't understand their odds of developing diabetes if they *didn't* get help. Prevention is difficult to routinize. It involves puncturing the illusion that all will be well if you change nothing, if you ignore the warning signs of mildly abnormal blood test results.

Scaling even gold standard Me programs such as DPP is difficult. Which is why when there is evidence that a particular Us program or policy is convincing (sugar taxes), even if not derived from a randomized trial, it can have population-wide effects.

* * *

Public health care practitioners have supported needle exchanges and HIV testing, instituted parenting programs to prevent disruptive conduct problems among children, promoted vehicle booster seats, aided school nursing services, encouraged home-based blood pressure monitoring, financed early education programs for low-income children, backed new therapies for juvenile offenders and their siblings, installed speed cameras on roads, endorsed medication adherence protocols in pharmacies, created special health programs for firefighters, assisted with animal control, to name a few of their activities. Age-old public health maneuvers such as water fluoridation are still needed in particular cities, and public health workers assist in these efforts. Public health workers educate the public about smoking cessation, distribute naloxone to reverse overdoses, inspect restaurants and tattoo parlors, track annual diseases such as influenza, provide flu vaccines and convince the public to use them at community health fairs, and lead teenage pregnancy education campaigns. Some of these public health activities (what your $286 per year goes toward, a bargain really) include the strict testing and comparison of protocols; most do not. The programs make sense; they seem helpful; recipients appreciate them. But they have not been proven effective through rigorous randomized trials.

We depend on natural experiments because the strict clinical trial testing of the great majority of public health activities is often not possible. Needle exchanges (the first on the list of harm reduction offerings above) are community-based programs in which people who inject drugs can turn in old, dull needles and receive free new ones so they don't have to share with friends whose needles may harbor infectious blood. To construct a randomized trial of needle exchanges is difficult. No one who injects heroin will sign up for a trial that randomly chooses whether they get to go to a needle exchange or not; potential participants already believe they know what's best for them to avoid acquiring HIV or hepatitis; they are likely already going where they want to go. You can't force someone to go to a needle exchange. Potential participants will refuse to be randomized. On the other hand, we can track, over time, how frequently a group of people who regularly seek needle exchange services acquires new HIV or hepatitis infections compared to a group that never visits an exchange, but we cannot "control" the use of such services easily.

Which is not to say that people who use heroin won't join *any* randomized trial. They may be sure about where they want to get clean needles but may be less sure about whether to try out the newest antidepressant medication that might help them be less fatalistic and perhaps find a way to quit heroin altogether. If asked to join a randomized trial comparing a promising antidepressant pill to a placebo (inactive sugar pill), some might join. These joiners might see the benefit of getting access to a new therapy, and getting it for free. They will not know whether they get the real medication or not until after the study ends, but if they like the idea of the possible benefit and are not put off by the known risks of this new medication (and there's always some risk of dry mouth, rash, etc.), they will enroll.

The policy question—Does making a needle exchange available reduce HIV across a population of persons who inject drugs? an Us question—can't be answered through a randomized trial. But the depression question—Will this new medication help Me be less depressed?— can. The policy question regarding needle exchange and HIV can be and has been answered in other ways, but the evidence in favor of needle exchange as a mode of prevention is far more circumstantial than the direct comparison and "proof" of a randomized medication trial.

As the psychology researcher Amos Tversky said, "It is sometimes easier to make the world a better place than to prove you have made the world a better place" (Michael Lewis, *The Undoing Project: A Friendship That Changed Our Minds*. WW Norton, 2017, p. 230).

But often we demand proof. And if randomized clinical trials are the only acceptable way to provide proof, we are limited to a Me world.

* * *

CHAPTER 7

PUBLIC HEALTH IS THOUGHT OF AS GOVERNMENT WORK, PRIMARILY FOR THE SAKE OF THE POOR

Let's come back to the tricky Me vs. Us conundrum about weight and unhealthy eating. A public health perspective of obesity offers a framework in which obesity is a social problem that stems from, and is cultivated by, a broad range of inequities. Some among us live in neighborhoods that don't have markets selling fresh fruits or vegetables. Some have low incomes and can't afford to bypass the middle supermarket aisles where the sales promotions for processed premade foods make for lower prices and where it's that much harder to fend off the sugary requests of our kids. A societal response to obesity then must include a thorough investigation of the structures that allow obesity to happen in the first place.

The social problem framework of obesity and its implications may not be relevant to many readers of this book. Why? Because it has nothing to do with you if you have enough money. You can

Me vs. Us. Michael D. Stein, Oxford University Press. © Oxford University Press 2022.
DOI: 10.1093/oso/9780197637562.003.0008

buy another diet book if the first doesn't work. You can buy better food. You can join a gym, or hire a personal trainer if that doesn't help. You can get better sleep, there's a pill for that. You can work around the high fructose corn syrup in the foods at the center of the supermarket. You believe you can control *your* life expectancy, like you can control *your* weight.

Tales of weight loss are personal success stories. Dieters talk about increased vitality and enjoying a healthy life. They talk about control: of hunger, of satiety. Dieters talk about private emotions such as shame, but also about satisfaction. Dieters create myths of self. A diet is not merely about weight loss: It's about being a better person, a better parent, making a new life. Dieting is Me focused, beyond health focused.

Taking a public health framework changes any self-improvement discussion to an Us discussion. By making the debate of social influences routine and system-focused—an admission that our food system is the product of agricultural and antitrust policies, political choices—a preventive health slant seeks a broader range of solutions.[1] Prevention moves away from our current approach of waiting for a full-blown manifestation of obesity and then bemoaning our ability to eradicate it.

* * *

If our life expectancy, the key gauge of our public's health, depends on first believing and then solving or mitigating the enormity of poverty and inequality, are we lost? It can feel that way. There are huge impediments to finding whole-cloth solutions: economics, geography, race, history. To make a dent, we must make society-wide arguments about the food we eat, the water we drink, the air we breathe, the buildings we sleep and work in, the schools we send our kids to, and the transportation networks we utilize. Public health is an argument for how to live. But changing any one of these factors that determine our health, that define the state of not getting sick to begin with, is like fighting a Hydra: Cut one off and two more grow back. We repeatedly need to find new responses to intransigent problems. Promoting health feels overwhelming.

Because of their scale, public health changes are necessarily slow. Improvements are difficult to see in real time, again making public health invisible. There are seemingly innumerable steps to produce change. If we don't ignore them completely, the size of the problems we are trying to address can frustrate us. We have two strategies to handle this frustration: First we turn to data and then to morality.

Fortunately, we are in the golden age of big data. Public health work proceeds from the assumption that public health is an aggregation of individual health, each given equal weight. Public health practitioners need to deliver programs in communities, and at the same time public health researchers can collect information about human lives into massive data sets in the hope that analysis of the aggregate will explain how to improve health for the individual.

Doctors, on the other hand, resist big data; they experience its limitations. Big data, once analyzed into averages, might offer a disinterested roadmap for a single patient's state of being but none of the vibrancy of the individual. Medicine looks away from the homogenizing aggregate-grip of big data and prefers a thousand tiny answers rather than one big answer. What emerges from the Me perspective is a case for the beauty of small data and its deliberate interpretation—a celebration of the infinitesimal, incomplete, imperfect, yet marvelously human details through which we wrest meaning out of the incomprehensible vastness of all possible experience. Big data provides only an impersonal vastness.

The work of public health is defined in part by the size of a problem. A problem affecting two people is not a public health issue. How about a problem affecting two in every town in a county (19,495 incorporated cities in the United States)? How about two in every county in the country (there are 3,143 counties)? What part of a population must be affected to make something a public health problem? Whatever number we decide, public health is *always* a distributional matter—what portion of the population in a town or county is healthy (or obese as we discussed previously). And public health workers are charged with considering the causes of that distribution.

When studying distributions, big data is the best guide to measuring and improving health that we possess, yet it loses to human detail. So public health turns to morality.

Public health is an argument about how to live, and the case is often made in the extreme. "Junk food is a form of violence perpetrated against the poor." Or as my colleague Lucas says, when I ask him how to improve the health of Americans, "We should reduce poverty." It sounds simple and clear. There is no disagreement with this statement among public health workers. "Should" is the language of virtue. Public health has an egalitarian promise. It pushes for utopia. And it is corrective: Justice arrives to right what has too long been wrong in the world. For our health.

But "should" is not an argument. The shared language of virtue cannot stand in for a unified approach. Addressing distribution issues such as poverty and inequality at scale is never simple and non-controversial; it requires government interventions.

* * *

Public health often offers directives. You should wear seat belts. You should get vaccinated. You shouldn't smoke. You should avoid unnecessary antibiotics. This command language, with its moral tinge, is at odds with the language of shared decision-making that has become central to the medical world; the patient decides after hearing from the doctor; together, the two come up with a plan of action.

In its use of "should," public health embraces an approach that can seem at odds both with notions of individual freedom and with medical norms. In the shared decision-making world of modern health care, doctors are meant to discuss options with patients, with the final health decision made by the patient, who may, in the end, make an unhealthy choice. But public health persists in suggesting courses of actions for the entire population, to be taken on a population's behalf. Why?

The answer is simple. Public health professionals know best for populations; individuals know best for themselves.

Let's use cigarette smoking as an example. Public health professionals are delighted that the prevalence of smoking has decreased from 50% to 16% in the past five decades. A future elimination of all tobacco use would be even better—the end of smoking would save millions more lives. Smoking's end, when it comes, will be caused by the same factors that drove smoking's decline—decisions made by public health professionals to improve the health of populations.

Shared decision-making is necessary at medical visits; clinical providers may be experts, but the best data about treatment may not apply to the patient in the office, and so her personal outcome is always in doubt. Hence, the patient can reasonably choose for herself among a number of uncertain options. But we can be much more certain about outcomes more generally when we are considering the health of populations. By any reasonable measure— longevity, cost to the health system, quality of life—smokers do worse than non-smokers. We can say this with certainty. After assembling incontrovertible evidence—in this case, of the hazards of smoking—public health providers try to universalize its application for the good of all. So, we tax cigarettes, we institute anti-smoking advertising campaigns, we eliminate indoor smoking, and we increase insurance premiums to smokers, all to create a healthier population.

Society entrusts public health to understand what is in the public good and to act on it. Therefore, when we know the healthiest answer, we should be relentless in seeking its implementation. It is up to society to decide if public health should or should not be in a position to flex its moral ("how we should live") muscles. When public health practitioners see opportunity to improve the public's health, which derives from the combination of evidence and public agreement, we should act, even in the absence of consensus.

When we use big data and bring in the word "should," we have naturally turned toward the power of government policy to improve health. We are searching for authority.

* * *

Public health struggles to find equitable and workable solutions to complex problems using three forms of legally binding public policy: legislation, regulation, and litigation. Legislation, also called statutory law, is created by elected representatives (e.g., from Congress, state assemblies, or city councils). Regulations typically add specificity to policies that are described broadly in legislation. Litigation refers to the body of public policy created through judicial opinions. Other policy tools, such as presidential or gubernatorial executive orders, are legally binding and bypass traditional legislative or regulatory processes, allowing for more rapid policy change.

Here's the standard public health list for developments that had the greatest impact on health and well-being during the 20th century: vaccination; motor vehicle safety; workplace safety and limits on child labor; decline in heart disease; recognition of tobacco as a health hazard; healthier mothers and infants (since 1900, infant mortality has decreased 90%, and maternal mortality has decreased 99%); safer food; fluoridated water; family planning; and control of infectious diseases such as cholera, typhus, polio, and measles.[2] What's notable is that nearly all of these accomplishments were linked to laws, including the Safe Drinking Water Act of 1974, the Infant Formula Act of 1980, the Pure Food and Drug Act of 1906, and the 1980 Occupational Safety and Health Act, and court rulings supporting crash standards, mandatory vaccination, contraceptive use, food labeling, fluoridation of public drinking water, and prohibition against advertising cigarettes on television and radio. Legal frameworks are supportive of, and necessary for, public health.

Federal agencies such as the Environmental Protection Agency, the National Highway Traffic Safety Administration, and the Department of Labor's Occupational Safety and Health Administration were not created explicitly to take regular legal actions expressly for the public's health, but they often do. It is difficult to think of a federal agency whose work does not affect health. These agencies help acquire information, monitor, provide enforcement, and allocate rights and duties. They write guidance documents that do not carry the force of law but provide answers when the law is unclear. They provide the legal framework and substantial funding for public health programs, although state and local public health authorities still implement the programs that provide the services outlined by policies.

Implementation determines a policy's success or failure. Policies that include clear, concrete definitions of the target population and detailed regulations to be applied are more likely to be successfully implemented than policies that leave such criteria subject to interpretation. For example, to be effectively implemented, a state law prohibiting the sale of sugar-sweetened beverages in schools should define which types of schools are subject to the law, criteria for defining a sugar-sweetened beverage, the date by which schools must comply with the law, and the sanctions that will be imposed on schools that do not comply with the law.

Equally, agencies not focused on health, such as the Federal Trade Commission, can also produce policies that indirectly undermine health. For instance, antitrust rule changes starting in the 1980s that permitted corporate mergers (as long as they didn't raise prices for consumers) propelled consolidation in the food industry. A small number of corporations now dominate each piece of the food economy. When we think of obesity, we understand that our food system is built upon a foundation of commodity crops—corn and soybeans—that are the building blocks for fast food, snacks, and soda. Our diet is dominated by highly processed food, and highly processed food is dominated by large corporations.

Our legislators are not always wise and ecologically aware altruists. Government officials can be myopic and self-interested. Government sometimes creates traps we cannot get out of.

* * *

Today, we're skeptical of government and its machinery. This skepticism comes in many shapes. Liberals have feared the military–industrial complex, and conservatives have feared an administrative state taking away their rights. High-profile initiatives such as limits on sales of jumbo sugary drinks or mask mandates to limit the spread of Covid-19 are seen by conservatives as interfering with personal autonomy and an overreach in the definition of public health threats, just as pornography "crisis" legislation is seen by liberals as religion eclipsing health.

For a generation, voters have moved to make government smaller; public health disinvestment is a symptom of disinvestment in governmental spending more generally—other than military spending, which, ironically, can be viewed as a kind of health prevention intervention. Such hesitance to unleash the federal government's purse and national coordination capabilities made it more difficult to deal with Covid-19 in 2020. But we should have expected nothing different. Our criticism of and lack of trust in government programs—the trope is that they are slow, wasteful, seemingly permanent—is widespread despite the facts (e.g., Medicare is far more efficient, administratively, than the hundreds of extant private sector insurance plans). The arrival of Covid-19 and the need for a federal response—to accelerate testing or mask-wearing rules or vaccination diffusion—might have put an end to the dispute about the need for strong government in the realm of public health. But trust in science depends on overall trust in government, which remains low. Individualists, Me-ists, value the primacy of personal goals over group goals. They value the regulation of behavior according to personal beliefs rather than social norms. Self-interest and self-reliance can foster innovation but undermine cooperation. Government, with its calls for collective action, can endanger individual liberties.

Our skepticism about government overreach encompasses our fear of public health as work overly entangled in social, economic, cultural values, that reaches too broadly, goes back to the origins of organized public health.

The British Public Health Act of 1848 provided a prototype for how we might improve public health.[3] It established both new laws about improving urban sanitary conditions and also formal public health infrastructures. The act established a general, central board of health, and in some places, local boards of health (mandated when the death rate of a district exceeded the national death rate; this criterion is perhaps worthy of resurrection). It was visionary in its focus on prevention and in establishing accountability for the health of the public.

But the central driver for the act was perhaps more economic than aspirational for a healthier population. Edwin Chadwick, the champion and master politician of this piece of legislation, knew that if he could improve the health of the poor, fewer people would seek relief from the government, ultimately saving money.

Public health is a practice and a process. It is not fast work today nor was it 170 years ago. The work of making a safer sewer system in London took two generations after Chadwick and many efforts.

Public health work is always a struggle. London's new system took a long time to finish building, but it saved hundreds of thousands of lives by direct protection from cholera and indirectly by serving as an example to other cities. Remaking the sewers required a process of reasoned reform but also evidence and argument and engineering. It was underground work, but, more important, it was government work.

The principle of public good and the process of public works became the same.[4] The complex methods of building public sanitation were inseparable from the abstract principle of the public good. Government's role was, after all, the protection of the public.

Chadwick understood that health was a function of society in operation, which meant public health was necessarily political. The public health perspective since Chadwick has included a corrective consciousness and argued that health depends on progress against poverty, which requires government—through expense and action, and through politics—to address inequalities. Public health has run up against the Protestant ethic that escape from poverty is a sign of good character and moral worth, and the false argument that if you give people more, they work less. Poverty has been seen as malign not only for what it is but also for what it does to health. Still, not everyone wants to be reminded of inequality or be told how to feel, think, and behave toward it. We don't want to have to choose sides.

CHAPTER 8

PUBLIC HEALTH IS MISSING HEALTH CARE'S PERSONAL STORIES

Medicine is about the body: its scars and story. It is about what one person does to another. You can show the body in a photograph, but what does a public look like? Or a community? How do you show the health of Harlem in a photograph?

Medicine is easy for us to understand because we have all experienced insults to our body. Public health injuries—air pollution inducing lung disease, diets predisposing to obesity—are more difficult to visualize but are no less real. Public health requires us to correctly interpret a wide range of information in front of us. We might see a map of Covid-19's distribution, for instance, with the note, "Each dot represents 500 deaths (infections)." On such a chart, nothing happens to a single person alone.

Medicine is country music in its specificity. Public health is oratorio, a choral work, long and large-scale. Public health pays attention at a different register. The public health "voice" faces, sings, outward as if on a stage. The medical voice only says, "That could be me." The medical voice is the one that is fundamental, the one we

Me vs. Us. Michael D. Stein, Oxford University Press. © Oxford University Press 2022.
DOI: 10.1093/oso/9780197637562.003.0009

experience every day talking to our children and friends through the power of the anecdote, of testimony, of confession, of witness. The public health voice says, "You should" or "You shouldn't." It castigates. It argues for reform. "You" means everyone.

* * *

It's almost always hot in July in Chicago, but during July 1995, thousands of Chicagoans went to emergency rooms dehydrated, cramping, exhausted, their kidneys failing. One by one they arrived, mixed in with patients suffering from the usual heart attacks, back pain, pneumonia, lacerations, skin infections, sprained ankles. Officially it's a heat wave when there are two consecutive days that exceed the 99th percentile of a county's usual seasonal temperature. Chicago was experiencing an extended heat wave. Severe heat stroke produces a core body temperature of nearly 106 degrees, producing tissue damage and distortion of blood chemistries. The ambulances arrived carrying patients who were confused, having trouble breathing. They carried patients to the 10 emergency rooms spread across the city so that each hospital received only a few overheated patients on any given day that July.

The disasters we think of occur in a single horrific event: a plane crash, a hurricane, an earthquake, a bombing. Tens or hundreds die suddenly, unexpectedly, with television coverage capturing the experience in real time. During the worst week of that month's unprecedented heat disaster, 739 Chicagoans above the norm of a typical July week died. No one knew the real "excess" death toll because many heat deaths were attributed to other causes. It was a catastrophe in slow motion, and mostly invisible amidst the usual summer illnesses. The city dwellers didn't arrive at hospital all at once. Maybe there were a few more than expected on any given day. But there was no special team mobilized to await them in emergency departments. These patients seemed to have little in common other than their body temperatures, and everyone knew it was hot outside.

The doctors treated them one by one. Chilled intravenous fluids. Ice packs applied strategically to the neck, axilla, groin, then spread all over the body; or better yet, a cooling blanket. More than half the patients required extended hospitalization. Each death had a physiological explanation: acute thermoregulatory failure.

During the month, there were more deaths than those from any single headlined disaster in memory. Even when patients survived the heat stress, a large number of those who made it to emergency rooms had permanent bodily damage; they would never recover the strength to walk again. Hundreds more died at home, never making it in for health care. It seemed like a whim of nature. These weren't occupational injuries; the deaths weren't occurring among agricultural workers or construction workers toiling outside all day. More than 1,000 people in excess of the July norm were admitted to hospital, but spread over 31 days and many facilities, the breadth or mortality was missed for a time. It wasn't until the morgues were overstuffed and meat-packing firms were providing refrigeration trucks to hold the bodies that it was clear the casualty count was extraordinary.

No single emergency room doctor attending to a patient or two on a particular shift and having only a few shifts per week could see the patterns or make the case for a widespread public problem. If you think in terms of individuals, you won't think in terms of patterns. There was a similar epidemiological delay for the same reason in the detection of lead poisoning in Flint, Michigan.

Eric Klinenborg, who has written forcefully about Chicago during July 1995, points out that the media also missed the pattern of deaths.[1] Commentators made assumptions that were importantly incorrect. Fatalities were "as varied as victims of a plane crash," one newscaster said. Those who died were "just like most of us," reporters wrote. In fact, the victims weren't random nor did they match the demographic characteristics of newspaper readers. Three-fourths were older than age 60 years. Men and Blacks were far more likely to die than women and Whites. The victims, it turned out, were most often elderly, poor, and isolated. In fact, the geography of vulnerability was a map of inequality. Social conditions had directed the deadliness of this heat wave. The reporters' language was inaccurate.

The reporting reflected our fascination with the medical world. Chicago reporters wanted stories of either heroic doctors or individual patients who had survival stories. They couldn't sell papers with a story about why hundreds of older citizens died alone in their apartments. A total of 170 bodies and their belongings went unclaimed postmortem because they had no known relatives. But newspaper and television reporters don't report about groups; they want to know what happened to a particular person. Newspaper reporters don't write about abstractions or big ideas. Why did so many die alone? Why did certain neighborhoods and groups experience disproportionate devastation? Why did social support systems designed to help the vulnerable fail? Reporters wanted to know: Where was the personal story within the larger story of the heat wave?

The Chicago heat wave was the perfect example of a public health story of anonymized lives. To tell the story required data collection. It required knitting together information from throughout the city and analyzing it by zip code and by neighborhood. It was the usual unappealing public health tale, slow to develop, complicated to tell, based in disadvantage, with few identifiable persons who had happy recoveries. It's no surprise that Chicagoans who weren't directly affected paid little attention.

In one sense, this was the story of those who never touched the health care system, who never saw a doctor before they died, as much as those who made it to emergency rooms. It was about social setting or what public health practitioners, epidemiologists, call a "risk environment," what I've called conditions and context. It was impersonal, a societal story. Neighborhoods of 65-year-old, poor Black men dying in their apartments alone. There was no uplift, no cure, and there were no transformational successes.

The Chicago heat wave is the perfect tale for those who think of the world in terms of and contingent on structure and context, and not in terms of a single person. It's the perfect story for readers who don't trust the individual medical story to explain the world, but who want the combined stories of a thousand persons. But most of us aren't interested in death statistics. Numbers are not the humans they are supposed to denote. Instead of statistics, we read obituaries. We want the personal stories, the anecdotes. We are moved by individuals and their urgencies. A few individual stories that become well known ("publicized") overshadow the many worth knowing.

* * *

The typical public health narrative is about the forces in our world that overtake Us. The typical public health narrative uses statistics to anchor the effects of such forces—Are the effects going up or down? On the other hand, a health care story (Me story) is about how one person feels in the grip of a particular force: illness. It's about the body's betrayal and pain and the sudden onset of emotions. It's about submission to illness and recovery from it, about resilience and joy, apart from numbers, almost apart from words. You could watch a video of the history of an individual's illness from beginning to end with the sound off and know the story.

The storytellers who care about public health have used Me narrative techniques to offer an Us tale. Giving public health *a story* can be done. But it's rare. And it's tricky. It often has a detective-tale element. Steven Johnson, in his wondrous book *The Ghost Map*,[2] provides the iconic account of the return of cholera to 1854 London, as investigated by John Snow, a celebrated anesthesiologist leading a double life as an outbreak investigator. Snow drew maps, knocked on doors in tough neighborhoods to interview residents about symptoms, and collected water use histories and samples, trying to find the cause of a diarrheal illness that was killing his neighbors at such a rate that the coffins were carried on top of hearses as well as inside.

We meet Edwin Chadwick of British Public Health Act of 1848 fame, believer in the miasma theory of infection (the odors and inhalations of unsanitary space spread disease). As sanitation commissioner of London, Chadwick understood that London had an excrement problem. He studied waste disposal and sewers, water pumps, and the underground pipes that were bringing, for the first time, running water into homes of the new metropolitan city that crowded 3 million people inside its 30-mile circumference. He essentially invented, or at least operationalized, the idea of public health as one of the roles of government: The state should directly engage in protecting the health and well-being of its citizens, particularly its poorest, using investment in infrastructure and prevention as recommended by health experts. The idea of government monitoring the water supply was revolutionary then, but it has lived on.

Public health thus began as social reform. Chadwick's major problem, a citywide sewer system, required engineering effort, but also the support of local boards that controlled the paving and lighting of streets, the building of drains, and the laying of new pipes. It required a master plan and Chadwick was a master planner. The Nuisance Removal and Contagious Disease Prevention Act of 1848, referred to as "the cholera bill," required sewer connections to existing structures; households could no longer dump their waste where they pleased. Nuisance, human waste, inspired the growth of public health.

The cholera tale has a second connection to public health, to one of its essential methodologies: contact tracing. Death rolls, "bills of mortality," had been around since the Plague in the 1600s when keeping records of who died was formalized. But only in the 1840s had London record keepers begun to include additional variables about those who expired: age, occupation, and, finally, cause of death. With these new statistical tallies, broad patterns of disease could be studied.

John Snow knew the addresses of those who had died and the families he wanted to interview to gather additional variables to test his theory. If cholera was waterborne, then patterns of infection would correlate with patterns of water distribution. He hypothesized that there had to be lines of connection from the individual pathology to the wider neighborhood. Where did the deceased get their drinking water? Snow shifted perspective from doctor to sociologist to statistician, the first representative of that admixture of professions that represent modern public health.

Public health methods helped sort out conflicting theories of the outbreak, suggesting an infectious agent rather than poisonous vapors as the cause of cholera. But the acceptance of a contamination theory centered on the Broad Street water pump was troubling and easy to resist; that pump had always been a reliable source of clean well water.

The irony of the story is that Chadwick routed sewage to the Thames River, which routed water back to Londoners' homes, just as John Snow was demonstrating that cholera was a waterborne illness.

The Chicago heat wave story could have happened any time (1995, 1975, 1925) in any city. To be a better public health story, it needed more context, it needed historical moment. It needed the eyewitness reports that newspaper assemble. It needed marquee stars playing detective roles.

Piecing the world of 1854 London together, *The Ghost Map* offers a taste of public health as a gumbo; everything's in there. The search for the cause of cholera provides a stew of variables and spices thrown into the pot. The smashing together produces a combined effect of taking up life expectancy, age-adjusted mortality, activities of daily life. Chadwick and Snow provided the star power, and 150-year-old investigatory documents and newspaper clippings were still available for perusal. The goal of any story is to make sure the reader never wants to look away. But a public health story makes room for the feeling of an entire community's uneasy disorientation. Public health is about culture and landscape and historical record. Its goals are cooperation, progress, equality, and stability.

In *The Ghost Map*, the patient-level story and the societal-level story become one. The Me in this public health story was a city, a community, which, by caring about a single thing—the "mortality area" of an epidemic in one neighborhood in London—acted or thought as one. The community assumed an individual voice that said, The Broad Street pump's handle must be removed.

* * *

PART 2

HEALTH INDIVISIBLE

IN Part 1, I argued that public health is distinct from medicine and that the individualism of medical thinking is costly in its cultural dominance. This divide between public health and medicine, I suggested, will be the pressing issue in the conversation about health and health care over the next years: Where should we allocate resources and attention? The answer will be an expression of our values.

The "patients" of public health are the communities that are cured when the handle is removed from the pump. The "physicians" of public health, the practitioners of the public health world who diagnose societal symptoms, include both local workers who make decisions on the ground and policymakers who make decisions on spending. Public health stories always have longer arcs than medical tales; they take years to unfurl. The drama during the past 2 years in the compacted time of a pandemic has been whether public health recommendations would be followed and the ensuing health care impact if they were not.

In Part 2, I argue that health care professionals, across thousands of private offices and clinics, need to engage with the social forces that shape health, becoming, in effect, public health practitioners. During their first medical school interviewing courses, doctors have traditionally been taught to take limited family and social histories. But more extended patient interviews, providing a wider focus on the socioeconomic drivers of health, on the forces that produce health—clean air, nutritious food, safe neighborhoods, income—can provide the perspective that lets doctors truly support health rather than just treat disease. I hope that clinicians can see themselves throughout their careers as being part of the community-based ensemble that generates peoples' health rather than playing a role only when patients are sick.

There is a good rationale for medical doctors, caring for individual patients, to work in the spirit of public health. Doctors, collectively, can change the public conversation by helping communicate the fundamental role of context in shaping health. Indeed, I have come to think that one of my jobs as a primary care provider is to entreat my patients to think of their environments—from the immediate surroundings of their home and behaviors of their family members to the walkability of the neighborhoods where they live, to broader policies such as state bans on indoor smoking—as crucial to their health. My secret mission is to add to my patients' ideas about self-change a new concern about community change, which may in the end bear on everyone's health.

* * *

Precision medicine promises that knowing an individual's gene sequence is valuable for efficiently targeting preventive strategies for that person (or persons, or specific subsets of a population) who will derive maximal benefit. Imagine a 50-year-old woman with elevated blood sugar readings who does not yet have diabetes. This patient could have her genome sequenced and have a tiny chip implanted to track her glucose level. Using minute-to-minute chip sensor data, she could modify her diet in a specifically prescribed manner. Or her future physician might begin a new molecularly targeted medication to prevent her from developing diabetes if her newly purchased diet book does not work or is too difficult to follow, or because she simply prefers a pill to fussing with what she eats.

But to know if such an approach works for this woman, or others like her, to realize improved diabetes prevention based on such a precision medicine approach, researchers would not only have to make new discoveries about "sugar control" genes (as of now, there is no single target) but also need to conduct randomized trials about the special diet or novel medication prescribed to prove their efficacy. Or we could skip the costs of performing new trials about genetic testing and personally designed diets and individually tailored medication, and enroll this woman with prediabetes into the Diabetes Prevention Program (DPP).

I'd rather imagine that we identified thousands of persons with prediabetes (through standard non-genomic tests) and connected them with available interventions so we could treat those people at once, and *now*.

But the National Institutes of Health (NIH), our primary funder of new health research, is increasingly focused on basic science and clinical trials for new treatments that promote individual (Me) health. The Centers for Disease Control and Prevention (CDC)—the likely funder of a DPP dissemination plan and the necessary funder of all Us programs reaching into neighborhoods, cities, and states—has an annual budget one-fifth that of the NIH. To increase longevity, the budget devoted to Us health must increase.

* * *

Our fascination with individual health is understandable. We all want to know: How do I make myself better? If we are true believers in self-improvement, the responsibility falls on the individual. This is the thinking that sets the stage for precision medicine. One objection to the DPP trial—the lifestyle intervention with changes in eating and increases in exercise meant to prevent diabetes onset—is that its outcomes do not tell you about *you*; population health comes from population data; you can't take a population (such as all the participants in a DPP roll-out) and make an individual prediction. Although ironically, this is exactly what the precision medicine companies are doing by picking a few genes that are associated with diabetes across a large database (population) of DNA samples and trying to apply this gene "score" to make a prediction about an individual. The entire precision medicine enterprise, which uses population genetic data to prognosticate or prophesize for an individual, is shaky, by which I mean imprecise. Yet doctors, responding to the requests of patients, offer it, and patients, who don't appreciate estimates or likelihoods, push for increasingly more personalization.

*　*　*

Health professionals have always fallen into the two basic categories of the medical "Me-ers" and the public health "Us-ers." The two traditions flow, respectively, from the anatomical study of the individual body and from the counting of multiple bodies during a cholera outbreak. The anatomists (Me-ers), going back centuries, dissected single cadavers dehydrated by diarrhea in narrow rooms and delivered detailed drawings and virtuosic theories of blood flow and brain power. The body counters (Us-ers), alternatively, traveled neighborhoods drawing street grids, looking for connections across time and space, concerned with social rituals such as well-water usage and shared living conditions. If medical care is a photograph (the body in agony, in extremis, in deterioration), public health is everything that happens before the photo is taken.

After Chadwick, the tradition of public health workers became one of passionate reform and the belief that such is necessary and possible through democratic measures, through organizations and activism, data, and public reasoning. Public health work became an incremental practice, if not an ideology, then a temperament and tone and way of managing the world, more than a fixed set of beliefs. Public health was ready to act on behalf of equity with a faith that life should be fair, or fairer, and not overdetermined by who an individual's parents were or how much money they inherited.

Medicine had its own political philosophy. It started with two people trying to make a contract. But it was more than a simple money-for-work trade. The patient asked for treatment, was willing to be a burden to this stranger. The doctor's way of thinking was not dependent on the characteristics of that stranger but, rather, on that person's need. The contract was mediated by an act of care.

I know from my own experience why medicine matters. What inspires us as embodied humans is not the slow progress of public health but, rather, the spontaneous moments of exaltation when our psoriasis melts away, when our cancerous growth is removed. To try to find meaning in slow-moving projects of dutiful public health reform can seem comical, if also earnest and well-meaning. Medicine's miracles open up a crack of light to eternity; we can live forever. Do we want to spend our newly found time pursuing a long obsession with housing or pollution?

As a Sunday morning walker across my city, out early to enjoy the deserted streets, as someone interested in neighborhoods and how people live, but who is also a primary care doctor, I toggle between the perspectives of public health and medicine, but their different scales often undo me. I picture myself beneath the branches of public health, in the discrete body, in the world of medicine, but also consider myself above, looking up into the impossibly detailed system of branches spread out over me—hardwood, towering, and far away—that includes all of us.

* * *

So far, I have divided explanations of health into two perspectives. One focuses on the social forces that drive groups of people toward poor health (e.g., poverty, racism), a structure of overt and unspoken rules that can only be addressed through a politics that takes up the perspective of public health. A second perspective looks at how as individuals we choose to resist these forces through our daily personal decision-making. Health can be viewed from either side of this so-called structure–agency distinction. We can fight obesity by urging politicians to advance policies that reverse poverty, one of the root causes for people turning to low-cost calorie-dense food. Or we can examine the motivations of individuals who are over-weight and figure out ways to persuade them to eat differently (of-fering elements of the DPP trial). Dieticians don't dispute the insight that reducing poverty helps bring down a population's weight, but they look at weight from a different perspective. The agent-based perspective is more useful to dieticians and doctors, who can't lift a neighborhood out of poverty but can change the way they advise a single patient to behave.

We understand that it is unfair for some people to be born into families with little money or to grow up in towns without a super-market and only a Dollar Store, with no public transportation to get them to a manufacturing job that has moved miles away, and we recognize that choices are constrained by these sorts of factors. But we are also skeptical when we are told that the choices of spe-cific individuals don't play *any* role in determining their particular weight fate.

The clean distinction between an Us (structure) perspective and a Me (agency) perspective is too severe. Neither perspective alone is fully convincing. We want to hold both perspectives, which to-gether better capture reality. There are state-level failures and per-sonal failures; the two perspectives are indivisible—both influence health and should be addressed together.

* * *

Envision a pasture shared by a community of cattle herders, open to all.[1] The pasture has an upper limit on the number of animals—let's say 100—that can graze and be well fed at the end of the season. Each herder receives a direct benefit when his animals use the pasture and suffers from the deterioration of the pasture if his or others' cattle overgraze. The 10 herders could cooperate, each allowing 10 of his cattle into the pasture. But each herder has a private strategy: *I will add one more cow to my herd and let it graze here.* Each herder is motivated to add increasingly more animals because he receives the profit from selling or slaughtering and bears only a share of the costs resulting from overgrazing that will result as increasingly more herders add cattle. The herder's strategy seems rational—that is, until the pasture has been ruined. At that time, his herd starves and he has zero profit because there are no other pastures nearby. Without negotiated rules for behavior in this common space, each herder may become locked into a selfish system that compels him to increase his herd without limitation in a world that is limited.

This is an old idea. Aristotle observes that "what is common to the greatest number has the least care bestowed upon it. Everyone thinks chiefly of his own, hardly at all of the common interest."[2] The cattlemen as a group do not necessarily keep an eye on the optimal economic level of grazing. Each man pursues his own best interest in a society that believes in the free use of public space.

This seems to confirm the idea that everybody's property is nobody's property. Wealth that is free for all is valued by no one. The herder who is foolish enough to wait for the equitable use of the pasture will only find that another herder has changed the rules. There is no assurance that the field won't be overused by others, leaving him without a field tomorrow. None of this would be a tragedy if there were endless grazing areas. But some common resources are limited.

Think of the water we drink. The pasture as a common good is a metaphor for the problem of pollution where a commonly held resource is misused without the knowledge or consent of its users. It's not only Flint, Michigan, that has had a water problem. Potentially contaminated water is delivered to 15% of Americans today with illegal and unhealthy concentrations of chemicals such as arsenic, radioactive substances such as uranium, or dangerous bacteria found in sewage.[3] Millions in the United States drink dirty water. When Covid-19 prevention required handwashing, in those regions where there was no clean water, environmental and public health failures intertwined.

It is difficult to get individuals to pursue their joint welfare as opposed to their individual welfare. The idea that groups would act in support of their group interests (Us) should follow logically from the premise of rational, self-interested behavior (Me). All members of a group would be better off if a shared objective were achieved (the pasture remains a food source, or a river remains potable, swimmable). Yet the possibility of a benefit for the group (Us) is insufficient to generate collective action. When one person (Me) exploits a public good (open pasture, available water), it undermines the incentive for a community to contribute voluntarily to the joint effort of keeping that good.

The perspective of quietly taking advantage of the efforts of other herders to keep their herd limited in number seems rational to the individual (Me). But it is not rational when viewed from the perspective of all involved because others then do damage to Us.

Unless there is coercion or incentive, or some other special device to make individuals act for the public good, the public's health is at risk because the temptation to free-ride dominates. We have established laws against corporations polluting rivers for profit, but we have not convinced enough individuals to stop polluting our air. We have ended up where no one wanted to be—in the midst of calamitous climate change, which is not rational when viewed from the perspective of Us.

In this case of greenhouse gases and the pollution of our air, the protection of a common good, of the public's health, requires centralized control. Individuals and markets have failed to set, monitor, or constrain bad behavior on this issue, which can kill us all. It requires government to establish and enforce rules, an authority that balances the Me and Us perspectives, for there to be any chance of success. We share a common future.

* * *

Water and air, which if polluted cause disease and death, are part of our pasture, the resources we share for our collective good. Libraries, parks, highways, fire departments, even national security are also public goods—common resources that need to be supported by collective investment so as to be accessible to all.

The reason they are public goods, rather than individual commodities, is that we have decided they are so fundamental to our well-being that they should not be entirely at the whim of private investment or market forces. Education, for example, benefits everyone; education is therefore supported by everyone as a public good.

Despite political challenges, public goods remain viable in the United States precisely because they are necessary for our safety and health. For 75 years, we have invested in road safety as a public good. We passed laws, created agencies, and educated people with the goal of creating a robust network of rules and safety procedures to reduce traffic deaths. Today, it would be difficult to find the politician who attacks road safety as an example of government overreach. This is because road safety laws are so clearly tied to our health.

Can we think of health itself as a public good?[4]

We all desire health, both for ourselves and for those we care about. We value health. We back up this with our money. We spend vast sums on health each year. Yet the overwhelming majority of this investment goes to health care, its technologies and delivery, rather than to improving the core social, economic, and environmental forces that shape health without which our health cannot flourish.

It remains tempting to think that health does not depend on our collective investment—that we can, as individuals, simply buy health for ourselves. We may believe that if we can just secure access to the best doctors and medicines, our health will be ensured. But is this really possible?

Can we be healthy without clean air and water, safe neighborhoods, safe roads, and supportive community networks? All of these conditions are themselves public goods, relying on our collective buy-in. Are the laws that protect us on the road really so different from the laws that keep us healthy in other parts of life? Health is arguably the quintessential public good, depending as it does on a range of component goods, all of which are shaped by common investment.

We must make the link between public goods and health as clear as the link between seat belts and safety. This has profound implications for our thinking about health versus health care, about how we feel about selective investments in infrastructure, in housing, in education, in transportation, in the environment. If we truly want to be healthy, we have no choice but to embrace public goods as the key to our collective health.

Our health is a public good. Move the words around and that sentence could also read: Our good is a public health.

* * *

At times, we understand clearly that health is a public good, benefitting us all and supported by our collective effort. An individual's health does not exist in isolation, as the Covid-19 pandemic showed. We understood as infections rose in particular regions that there were not enough resources, not enough ventilators or intensive care unit beds. It was horrifying to contemplate running out of either. Our private enterprise system and our social net sharing system both activated. The virus was its own grim force, organizing us. The commons, our health, had to be protected.

We made individual choices based on how they might affect our housemates, our neighbors, our workplaces, our cities, our states. Even if each of us was paranoid and, while still caring most of all for ourselves, we understood our health concerns were clearly linked with others. We self-quarantined when we felt our responsibility to others. We made radical changes; we stayed inside; we kept apart where we could. We communicated our caring in these ways. There was no perverse logic in Me competing with Us. Selfishness and altruism coexisted, or became the same, at least early in the pandemic, before vaccination became abundantly available and many refused to be vaccinated.

Public health and health care perspectives merged during the first year of Covid-19. We integrated containment and care. We surveilled for new cases, but we also had a way to receive oxygen and intravenous fluids and medication if we needed them. Disease control and good medical care were two sides of the same coin. Doctors lived in the occupied city of sickness; outside, health happened.

* * *

With the Covid-19 pandemic, public health and health care perspectives overlapped. But there are other health issues where the two outlooks need to meet. One of the terrible and continuing health threats is the emergence of bacteria not killed by any standard antibiotics. The majority of doctors who treat infectious diseases in the United States report having seen an infection that did not respond to any treatment. Like coronavirus, for which we had no cure, bacteria resistant to antibiotics can spread easily from person to person and from country to country. Like Covid-19, these bacteria can spread silently, asymptomatically. Antibiotic resistance does not mean the body has become resistant to antibiotics; rather, bacteria have become resistant to the antibiotics designed to kill them.

Antibiotics underpin every aspect of modern medicine. We use them to treat symptomatic infections and, if administered before cesarean sections or joint replacements, to prevent infections from occurring after surgery. Antibiotics save lives, but any time they are used, they can produce resistant bacteria. The rise of antibiotic resistance was inevitable with the use of antibiotics. Bacteria change when they are exposed to drugs; most die, but some survive and multiply, reducing the effectiveness of those drugs they have outlived. Penicillin was released for public use in 1941. By 1942, the first penicillin-resistant bacteria were seen. Antibiotic-resistant bacteria thrive in hospitals and medical facilities, putting all patients—whether they're getting care for a minor illness or major surgery—at risk. But one doesn't even need contact with the health care system to become infected. Because anyone can ingest foodborne bacteria—from spinach or undercooked chicken—that cannot be treated, antibiotic resistance is a widening public health problem. Approximately 35,000 Americans die each year from an untreatable bacterial infection.

What is the Me perspective on resistance? We all try to prevent infections; when we get a cut or scrape, we clean it. Similarly, we should try to prevent resistance by using as few antibiotics as possible. The dominant cause of resistance is antibiotic overuse. More than 270 million antibiotic prescriptions are handed out in pharmacies each year, and at least 80 million are thought to be unnecessary, given for infections such as bronchitis or sinus and ear infections that will get better on their own. Therefore, individuals can limit the problem by talking with their health care providers whenever a prescription is written. Each of us should ask, "Do I really need this medication?" But once initiated, resistance can be mitigated by taking the full prescription as written. That is, don't stop medications because you feel better; don't share pills; don't keep leftovers for some future infection. But avoiding antibiotics is the best course; your overuse puts me at risk because bacteria share resistance with one another, live on our skin, and spread across the population when we touch doorknobs, supermarket baskets, counters.

What is the Us perspective on bacterial resistance? First, we need to recognize that our arsenal of antibiotics is not sufficient to guarantee today that we could manage any large outbreak tomorrow of any of a dozen different resistant bacteria that we know exist in our environment. Second, as a public health matter, we (our hospital and health department laboratories) need to track the spread of resistant bacteria so we have a chance to treat appropriately with particular antibiotics if one is identified in a sick patient. If a patient survives an antibiotic-resistant infection, it often requires early detection, an extended hospital stay, and costly and toxic experimental alternatives to the usual treatments. Third, and here again we draw lessons from Covid-19, we need to plan ahead for worst-case scenarios. We must remain aware that medically important antibiotics are given to food-producing livestock every year and such usage can cause antibiotic resistance in humans when these animals are eaten. Unfortunately used for animal weight gain without prescriptions from veterinarians, and given for unlimited durations, the presence of antibiotics in our food supply is putting us all at risk. As a public health measure, we need tight regulations to ensure that antibiotics are only used for carefully defined purposes. Fourth, because microorganisms will evolve to resist every existing drug—and every new one developed—we need to continue to develop new antibiotics. If we allow the pipeline for new medications to dwindle, the price won't be just in dollars but also in lives. Prescribers should prescribe new antibiotics as sparingly as possible to preserve their effectiveness for as long as possible, which reduces the enthusiasm of drug companies to invest in medications that are best if used the least. Incentives for new antibiotic research and development must be put in place. Medication stockpiling should be happening now (just as we needed personal protective equipment and ventilators when the time came).

The *U.S. National Action Plan for Combating Antibiotic-Resistant Bacteria* divides its report into urgent threats, serious threats, and concerning threats, depending on how few options there are to treat the life-threatening infections caused by these bacteria.[5] In a perfect world, we would always have new antibiotics to fight emerging antibiotic-resistant infections, ready to use when a resistant-bacteria crisis as widespread and unexpected as the one caused by the virus we call Covid-19 strikes. We can see it coming. We don't want to have to ask: Why weren't we prepared?

* * *

Hepatitis B and C are viral infectious diseases that affect millions of Americans. Left untreated, they cause liver cirrhosis and death. Both infections are preventable by reaching out to those at risk and teaching prevention behaviors, and such programs fall in the domain of public health. Yet Congress has historically funded viral hepatitis prevention programs at only $1 for every person,[6] based on the number estimated to be living with these conditions. Prevention programs could not exist, let alone be successful, on federal grant funding alone.

The first step in any viral prevention program is testing (again think of Covid-19); we need to know who's at risk and who's already infected and needs treatment. Widespread testing is both a form of surveillance and a form of diagnosis. Public health and health care have struck a deal. Public health program directors, rather than using their limited funds, have asked for testing to be paid for by health insurers. Why do public (Medicaid) and private (Blue Cross) insurers cover what could otherwise be considered public health testing? Because government policies have mandated it.

The same dynamic is true of HIV and sexually transmitted disease programs, which similarly rely on a mix of federal grant funding to public health agencies and insurance reimbursement for testing. I am not suggesting that this system is ideal, but cobbling together whole programs out of a patchwork of payers is what has enabled a viable public health response to viral hepatitis, albeit a woefully underfunded one.

The same cost-sharing arrangement has been created for providing childhood vaccines. The CDC invested millions in a project to help local health department immunization administrators learn how to bill health insurers for vaccination services (because vaccine coverage in those programs is mandatory) for their insured patients.[7] Leveraging these funds from health care insurers, public health departments were then able to target use of limited federal public health dollars to cases in which no public or private health insurance was available. Public health resources focus on targeted community-based vaccination while insurance picks up vaccine coverage in health care settings.

Obviously, a vaccine program launched in tandem with ensuring universal insurance coverage would be more efficient and comprehensive. But that's not how our system works currently.

Just as public health programs rely on insurance mandates to expand routine screening for HIV and viral hepatitis, mandates for insurers had to include (without cost-sharing) the range of Covid-19 testing that individuals needed to stay healthy and that the nation needed to manage the pandemic.

The amount of funding for testing, contact tracing, and surveillance that went to state and local health departments for Covid-19 was unprecedented in its scale and helped mount state and local public health responses to the pandemic.[8] But such departments had been underfunded for years, and their workforces were unprepared to cover vital prevention services during a public health and economic crisis.

* * *

There was a moment when public health and health were almost unified.

In 1916, the idea of a national health insurance plan first arose as the next great step in social legislation during the Progressive Era of widening the role of government. It was viewed as an opportunity to reorganize medical care. Its advocates envisioned groups of salaried physicians and nurses working under the supervision of local health departments, an arrangement that was meant to encourage preventive medicine and thereby "prove to be the greatest public health measure ever enacted."[9] At that moment, the surgeon general, head of the Public Health Service, was also the leader of the American Medical Association, the professional association of physicians, naturally linking the two fields. The first order of business, one advocate pronounced, would be to keep the death rate low: "Some day the care for the public health will be organized ... as a public service."

But health care never became more centrally directed, or driven by a public health perspective. The moment passed. Private medical practice surged, and the free market attacked the idea of widening federal programs. The delivery of health care, without united doctor groups or hospital systems and with its patchwork of insurers, was not in 1916, nor at any time since, about scaling interventions to reach entire communities, cities, and states. Because its perspective is focused on the care and survival of individuals, health care planning as we know has been fitful, hyperlocal, episodic, and necessity-driven.

* * *

I started this book suggesting that life expectancy, or the expectation of living 70 years, was a reasonable metric for judging the health of a group of people. But admittedly, mortality is a narrow way of defining health. We could just as easily count healthy days or the number of those who are sick across a population, as well as tabulating deaths. There are other health metrics: self-ratings of quality of life and disability-free years, for instance. As our lives have been extended, there has been a shift from illness threatening our longevity to poor health preventing our enjoyment of life, lowering productivity and reducing prosperity. Indeed, the impressive increase in longevity has not been matched by improvement in living in good health with a sense of well-being; today, we are living a greater proportion of our lives with disabilities and chronic diseases. On average, the last 15–20 years of life are lived in poor health, most often with limitations in mental and social health.[10] Again, the most deprived groups, our most impoverished neighbors, fare the worst in disability-free life years, yet another inequality. The gap between high- and low-income people in *healthy* life expectancy is double that of life expectancy. Whatever the health metric, we are left with the question of what factors contribute most to creating and preserving health. We might choose to invest more in the components more likely to make us healthy.

Some have tried to force the list of contributors to health to add up to 100%.[11] The County Health Rankings attributes weights of 40%, 30%, 20%, and 10%, in order, to social and economic factors, health behaviors, clinical care, and physical environmental factors that impact a community's health. These percentages have very little basis beyond "expert" opinion; they are guesses, value judgments. It is difficult to be more exact or to point to sources for these estimates. But if taken seriously, based on this metric it would be societally rational to invest primarily in ways to influence social and economic factors that as we've seen can secondarily improve individual health behaviors.

The problem is that long-life expectancy follows from the interaction of multiple causes. Heart attack deaths are related to rates of diabetes, which are related to rates of obesity, which are associated with a variety of societal policies advertising unhealthy food in low-income neighborhoods, where there are no parks to exercise, which as I've described are related to persistent poverty and intergenerational disadvantage. If we had to attribute weights to these contributors to heart attacks, how would we make them add up to 100%? What percentage should be attributed to health care, where the heart attack victim might or might not ever arrive, where it may be too late for effective medical interventions—surgery, stents, medication—to postpone death from heart disease? These advances may not even be accessible to a population that lacks insurance (a public health issue). Perhaps this is why "clinical care" contributed only 20% to the health of a community as rated by experts.

Do we ask health care providers to have a role in addressing diabetes and obesity to prevent heart disease to begin with? Of course. But given the growing prevalence of these conditions, doctors haven't been very successful. Health care planners have barely invested in initiatives such as DPP.

A public health perspective suggests DPP could be scaled but that it needs to be supplemented by attention to the conditions and contexts that work against prevention of heart disease (poverty, the price of fresh food, the price of cigarettes), that inform the behaviors that drive heart disease (eating, smoking). And then there's the contribution of one's genetics to heart disease, a driver of outcomes that is perhaps beyond the influence of either health care or public health.

A health contributor ranking list is not meant to be read negatively as a litany of blame. Rather, by displaying the concatenation of causes that contribute to health, we can see that interventions to *improve health* must occur at many levels because of the interactions between these causes. But which interventions? To choose the most powerful interventions, we would want to know not only how much a factor affects health but also how much we can modify that factor, and by what means. Again, there is no weighting system that clearly tells us how much to spend on public health and how much on health care. But if social and economic factors drive 40% of our health, public health should receive a greater share of our health improvement dollars (more than the 3% it currently receives), even if public health practitioners can rarely do randomized trials of complex policies that might offer the clearest direction.[12] On the other hand, the health care system is not doing its best to provide the "best" answers either; less than 0.1% of the $2 trillion spent per year on health care is devoted to evaluation of which interventions work and which don't.[13]

Forcing known factors to sum to 100% provides a false sense of security that we can draw a full picture of what drives health and where to invest. Much of health isn't explainable or modifiable by any means we know or are likely to discover soon. We should be humble about how much we can improve health. A clearer understanding of what we know, and what we don't know, is a better path to ensuring that our investments truly pay off.

* * *

The United States spends nearly twice as much per capita on health care as other developed countries, yet our health as a nation is mediocre—at every income level we are less healthy than Europeans and live shorter lives, as I've noted previously. One explanation for this paradox has centered on an understanding that health is dictated by more than health care—that social factors, conditions and context, matter far more for a population's health.

The United States spends about the same per capita as European countries on social factors (e.g., unemployment benefits, work training programs, housing, pensions, and education). But because the United States spends so much on health care, it has a far higher health care to social care spending ratio compared to European countries (or Australia or Canada). This ratio might be a better measure of how much we societally "value" each. The ratio suggests that we believe that more health care compared to more social factor spending might improve health most. In the United States, for every dollar spent on health care, only 60 cents is spent on social services, whereas in most countries, for every dollar spent on health care, two dollars is spent on social services. If we were to follow the County Health Rankings, which attributed greater weight to social and economic factors (40%) and lesser weight to clinical care (20%) in impacting a community's health, our ratio should probably be reversed.

Again, as a nation we seem to be committed to spending considerably more on medical treatment than on public health. A defender of that position might ask doubtfully: Does social policy spending actually *cause* better health? Causation is difficult to prove. The evidence is circumstantial but consistent: Particularly for those with the least income, with the least room for further depletions, policies directed toward them (earned income tax credits, etc.) are helpful. And compared to other developed countries, the United States has the highest rate of poverty; a large swathe of the population needs such assistance. But individually, the patient who receives curative medical treatment is sincerely grateful; Me money always feels like a good buy to the person who gets a good result.

* * *

If health care and public health come to share available financial resources more equally, and if government is the largest spender, then we keep returning to the key question: What are the specific large-scale interventions that have the largest effect on health? These could be in the domains of health care (treatments) or in other areas that principally target social needs (e.g., housing or education, or perhaps income, which affects both housing and education) but that may also have health effects. Historically, interventions directed at social domains don't typically measure health outcomes. Food insecurity or job insecurity have been shown to compromise health, but when developing action plans to improve either, health is not the primary goal of the intervention—food and jobs are. Higher education interventions (e.g., free college tuition) often report only the cost per student enrolled, but not any long-term health benefits. Tax policies measure revenues, the financial benefit that a policy provides to its recipients and the policy's net cost to the government: but the writers of tax policies never directly concern themselves with health.

But if you believe at this point that poverty (or income more generally) is central to health, then every governmental tax and spending policy that affects poverty should be considered a health policy. These policies might be divided into four domains: social insurance (e.g., health, unemployment, and disability insurance), education (e.g., preschool, kindergarten through grade 12, college, and job and vocational training), taxes and cash transfers (e.g., tax rates and earned income tax credit), and in-kind transfers (e.g., housing vouchers and food stamps). You can see why the remit of public health is expansive, why my colleague Lucas said, "Public health is everywhere."

Let's look at two specific policies—one that sits at the intersection of health care and public health is health insurance, meaningful to the lives of individuals, and one that can reach millions. Since its creation in 1965, Medicaid has been critical for improving access to health care for the poor. The United States had for many years ranked low in infant survival compared with other developed countries. Originally, Medicaid coverage for pregnant women was limited to a subset of the indigent population. Starting in 1981, Medicaid became available to a widening group of previously uninsured pregnant women who were too often delaying prenatal care until late in pregnancy because of fear of the expense of medical visits.[14]

The estimated cost of insuring an additional woman through this new rule was $3,473. An increase in health insurance coverage for pregnant women corresponded with reductions in low birth weight and infant mortality, a clear health effect (life expectancy changed for newborns). Moreover, by following these women and children for decades, researchers found positive impacts on children's future earnings and health for those whose mothers gained Medicaid eligibility during pregnancy. Some researchers estimated that a one percentage point increase in parental eligibility leads to a reduction in future hospitalizations of 0.24% when their children are aged 19–32 years, a 3.5% increase in college attendance, and an 11.6% increase in earnings for their children. By the time children are aged 36 years, the estimates suggest the policy has paid for itself. By the age of 65 years, the government recoups an additional $6,114 in tax revenue from these children's earning over this period, for a total of $10,023. The upfront cost of $3,473 led to a long-term net government surplus of $7,014. The policy evaluated here expanded health care opportunities to parents and children and, importantly, *did not make anyone worse off* as broad policies sometimes do.

In a second example, Chetty and colleagues studied the long-term impact on economic self-sufficiency of the Moving to Opportunity (MTO) experiment of 1994, which gave vouchers and counseling to assist low-income persons living in public housing and interested in moving to better neighborhoods. Chetty et al. documented that moving to a less poor neighborhood significantly increased later-life earnings for those children who moved before they were 13 years old.[15] The policy had little effect on the later economic outcomes of the parents, or even of children who were older teenagers when enrolled, but the effect on younger children was dramatic. By their mid-20s, their annual income had increased 31%. Where you live matters. Health, not the primary interest of program planners, was not measured for these children, but we know that health—the likelihood of living to the age of 70 years, longevity—usually tracks with income.

The Medicaid example and the MTO experiment are illustrations of a clear and persistent pattern in public policy: Direct investments in our youngest children yield large value. There is an enormous "bang for the buck" associated with a range of programs for children, from early education to child health insurance and college expenditures.

Of course, if we were to choose one policy to maximize our health right from the start, we would choose that everyone is born to high-income, well-educated parents who live in good neighborhoods. Luck in life's lottery is not really a policy, however.

* * *

Obviously, it's possible to do good for individuals. This is the medical approach. The MTO experiment demonstrated that families matter as the drivers of one's educational prospects. As a child, the patterns for your life are firmly (although not irrevocably) set. How much attention are your parents paying to you? This of course depends on how much money they have and how much time they can spend paying attention to you. What kind of education are you getting? The kind of college you go to is determined by the extent to which you had the right mentoring and whether you completed high school. Along the way, you become literate about what behaviors you need to have to promote your health.

The next level up from the individual and her family is the neighborhood, which many argue is the essential unit of social change and the one likely to be most available to public health efforts, where policy can most powerfully affect the structures or systems that influence lives.

I cannot say it too many times: Place matters. The average American lives 18 miles from their mother. The typical college student enrolls in a college 15 miles from home. On Facebook, 63% of "friends" live within 100 miles of each other. Within this small radius of social ties, behavior is highly contagious. We shape one another's behaviors. Neighborhood networks produce outcomes: suicide, obesity, smoking. On April 1, 2010, 44% of low-income Black men in Watts, California, were incarcerated.[16] Only 6.2% of men with similar incomes in Compton, 2.3 miles away, were incarcerated. In Klinenborg's Chicago heat wave analysis, there were more than six times the deaths in north Lawndale than in south Lawndale, demographically similar neighborhoods, separated by a road.

What makes a neighborhood a healthy place to live? It's not only that it has a hospital and an emergency room. There are other important structures: a grocery store, a fire station, a playground. But what else does it need? The key ingredient may be thickness of community bonds, more people checking up on each other. More places for neighbors to meet. More clubs, more community centers. These are not easy attributes to measure, but they are critical.

If we want to improve health, policymakers, government, or philanthropists who typically choose one kind of program or service to fund or promote—park creation, the installation of supermarkets to end food deserts—should instead look to bolster neighborhoods based on local needs. Neighborhoods have a hidden complexity, and we have to change many things in a single neighborhood all at once to make residents healthier.

* * *

The NIH, the United States' principal funder of biomedical research, puts its monies primarily toward basic science and randomized trials focusing on treatments that promote individual health, rather than toward studies of neighborhoods. We spend considerably more on research that has to do with the words "gene," "genome," or "genetic" than with the word "prevention." The proportion of NIH-funded projects with the words "public" or "population" in their title, for example, has dropped by 90% during the past 10 years.[17] The hope is that genetics will point us toward treatments susceptible to personalized intervention.

Genetic insights already touch aspects of prevention, which is typically the domain of public health. Hereditary breast and ovarian cancer syndrome and Lynch syndrome are common genetic conditions associated with premature death from cancer that is preventable. The same is true of familial hypercholesterolemia, which leads to heart disease. In aggregate, an estimated 2 million people in the United States have one of these conditions, and most are not aware of their risk. Identifying such patients at risk, we can prevent the development of certain conditions. Screening newborns for genetic illness is already the largest established precision medicine–public health program in the United States, prevention raised to a population level. Health care meets public health indivisibly. Health 2.0.

But so far this alignment of health care and public health interests applies mostly to newborns. As a country, we have poured money into identifying increasingly more genes, but these discoveries have not led us to more effective, widespread treatments for individuals with common conditions. And with less than 1.5% of total biomedical research funding devoted to implementation of effective prevention programs, too little attention is paid to the translation of scientific discovery to effective prevention policies that will improve our health.[18]

Historically, improvements in longevity for a nation have come from improvements in economic conditions. Longevity is also driven by programs that address an entire population, such as mass immunization or tobacco control, or with Covid-19, more simply, wearing masks.

* * *

Views on how to respond to the Covid-19 pandemic became increasingly polarized during the first summer of the coronavirus in the United States. The decision to wear a mask was seen as a partisan or ideological issue. On one side were those in favor of sacrificing personal liberties in exchange for containing the virus' spread. A mask was the indication that you took the pandemic seriously and were willing to make a personal sacrifice to save others' lives. On the other side were those who believed a mask was an infringement on where people could go and what they had to wear. They believed the mask was an overreaction; those most willing to misrepresent the data suggested that masks were not protective and that the mounting evidence demonstrating masks' effectiveness at limiting the spread of Covid-19 was inadequate. This split may have run along political party lines, but it most certainly was also a matter of perspective: Us (mask wearers) vs. Me (mask refusers). Our views of health were divided.

In early April 2020, the CDC issued its first recommendation that Americans wear "cloth face coverings" (surgical masks were still in short supply). Face coverings were not usually for personal protection as most wouldn't offer protection from possibly inhaling the coronavirus. But in situations in which social distancing is more difficult to do, such as a workplace or grocery store, a mask reduced the ability of an asymptomatic infected person to spread the virus. "With the masks, it is going to be a voluntary thing," President Trump said at a White House briefing on April 3. "You can do it. You don't have to do it. I am choosing not to do it. It may be good. It is only a recommendation, voluntary."

Initially, there was little evidence supporting how much widespread community mask use would affect the spread of Covid-19. Previous randomized trials for other respiratory illnesses were limited. But within 4 months the data became clearer as a natural experiment took place. Some state governments set mandates around mask use in public whenever the social distance could not be maintained, whereas others were more laissez-faire. The policies varied in their strictness and consequences of noncompliance. Twenty-one days after signing such executive orders or directives, the 15 states with mask mandates had 2% less daily Covid-19 growth than non-mask-use states, averting an estimated 230,000–450,000 new infections.[19]

As Covid-19 continued to spread, the evidence of masks' preventive effectiveness grew. Yet the wearing of masks never became a norm in parts of America because the impulse to think collectively (Us) about disease was never a dominant perspective. We had no public health norms, and no experience with serious epidemics. Mask refusal was a sign of tribal affiliation and the tribe was called Me.

* * *

Health has always been a predictor of work opportunities. One of the principal lessons of the Covid-19 era has been that a healthier population leads to a healthier economy, benefitting all rather than just the most deprived. As millions of Americans were sickened, life was interrupted. The most affluent maintained their incomes (and health) working from home, but their favorite stores, theaters, and restaurants were closed and their children were home from school. Elective surgeries were canceled and emergency rooms were dangerously overloaded, delaying care for non-Covid-19 patients. *Let everyone decide for themself*—regarding vaccinations, regarding mask wearing—did not produce widespread safety. Health was recognized as a communal experience, not merely a private one; each of us was vulnerable to Covid-19 (although inequities were quickly apparent). Health was viewed more than ever before as a shared value, a community asset. Still, it was the poor, and in particular Black Americans, who were at greater risk of severe Covid-19, patterned on underlying disproportionate morbidity, stemming from lifetimes of structured racism and disadvantage. Post-Covid-19, we will unfortunately again have to ask if it is worth investing in a healthier population (and not just an ever-more-expensive health care system), even though we now recognize that good health improves the life chances and economic fortitude of individuals and communities.

* * *

Having now lived through Covid-19, there seems then little argument that when Covid-19 arrived, public health was underfunded. Public health system funding had decreased per population during the past 30 years due to a combination of budgetary decisions and population growth. Most U.S. states spent less than $100 per person on public health, and most local governments spend more on policing than on health. The public health system entered the pandemic down more than 20% of its workforce capacity.[20]

The public health system in the United States remains decentralized. Despite the CDC's preeminence, public health authority belongs not only to the 50 states but also to thousands of counties and municipalities. The federal politicization of Covid-19 found easy entry through this rickety scaffold, which in its structure necessarily produces intergovernmental conflicts, delays and gaps in data collection, and undermines the authority of local public health officials.

Decentralization affected all aspects of the Covid-19 response. Immunizations, for example, could be provided by a local health department in one region but by other entities (e.g., pharmacies) in a second region. Thus, immunization, considered by many an essential public health program, was not rolled out according to a national model.[21] If it had been, could we have vaccinated more people, faster?

In addition to the roles of the public health system, it is aspects of American society that lay outside the scope of public health department activities which made the U.S. population susceptible to the rapid community spread and mounting deaths of Covid-19. Health departments do not focus on the provision of better elder care or on structural inequalities—poverty, a long history of racial discrimination—that produced high vulnerability among essential workers, two key constituencies that drove the U.S. epidemic. If we'd spent more on public health, if we'd invested more in the preventive conditions of health, would we have been more prepared for and responded more robustly to

Covid-19? Partisan goals, the politicization of vaccines, and the mistrust of institutions may have undermined even a prepared public health system in 2020.

Did the arrival of Covid-19 finally change the way we think about public health and the historical divide between public health and medicine? We need to think about the full scope of the forces that create health—both when we are in a pandemic and when we are not. It will require constant attention to and investment in ways to improve the foundational drivers of health to truly mitigate the risk of a next pandemic, no matter the strength of our medical systems. But public health has historically not been empowered (or funded) to tackle these issues and so we will remain vulnerable to contagion.

* * *

Although I believe that the public health solutions, in the end, are policy solutions, these arise only when society is paying attention. But the fundamental concept, the need to change societal incentives from sickness cure to keeping health, seems indisputable. Simply stated, the medical care system needs to embed public health thinking and practice. Doctors can move their health systems to insist on screening all patients for and creating interventions around the most tangible social drivers of health—food, shelter, and income. No one more than a doctor is aware of the moral and social resources that people draw on to survive and transform their conditions of life. In my office, I can set an example for this new tradition of paying attention to the drivers of public health that influence individual health, by trying to attend to these conditions as one would for any other patient symptom.

When I ask a patient in my office, "Do you ever have difficulty making ends meet at the end of the month?" the conversation opens into the concerns and priorities of public health. We talk about bills and budgets, rent and income and expenditures, and skipping medication doses to save money. We talk about jobs and school and debt. We talk about how poverty drives stress, chronically, daily, which leads to bad health outcomes.

For many people, chronic diseases are a product of one's past. I talk to patients about how never having had much money growing up led to eating lousy food and putting on weight as a teenager, which led to a sedentary job, and finally to diabetes. There are many causal pathways to illness, not all of which need to involve self-blame. The medical history and the public health history meet at the social history. Doctors need not concentrate only on a checklist of physical and emotional symptoms or on the select part of life history that a patient does alone—eat, sleep. I can consider the symptoms produced by systems: Does this patient live in a broken building or eat in an unclean kitchen or work installing insulation in attics? Who does she spend time with? Medicine and public health first meet in the realm of social relations.

By the time anyone sees a doctor, they are playing catch-up. Understanding how the context of a medical problem contributed to that problem allows my patients to recognize that they have a symptom that might have been prevented. Which means, as they think of ways to improve their own health, they also think about their children's health and new means of health promotion for their families.

My job becomes, in part, to entreat patients to think of their environments as drivers of their health. I want my patients to appreciate, for example, that we collectively push for indoor smoking bans—limiting the freedom of some to smoke anywhere—because we want to avoid cancer risk, and we don't want our asthmatic friends sickened by secondhand smoke. I am not trying to make everyone into an activist and of course most people—whose lives are already filled with obstacles and demands—have limited bandwidth to take on these larger issues. But some do.

* * *

Although I started this book with the claim that health care and health are competing interests, I am ending with what should now be clear: Individual and public health are inseparable. We need to recover and sharpen our sense of health, based on a reverent appreciation of both perspectives, of humankind, one by one and all together.

The objective of public health, then, is not only health but also the constant announcement about the need for health and the threats to health. In this way, public health seems unattainable and therefore both beckoning and burdensome, aspirational as a perspective. Public health is political (being part of a group, citizenship) as well as personal (taking into account our identities, with the understanding that our health today is a product of our past).

"We're in this together" was a phrase often heard during the pandemic. A common identity at risk gave us a reason to care about and help each other. Our identity became that of a group that could get ill. We were individuals within a collective. We acted altruistically because we were selfish. Covid-19 has taught us that heath is built when people make promises to one another to solve a common challenge. But to hold one another accountable and sacrifice together requires a sense of social cohesion, trust, mutual respect, and an admission that the inequities existing in health care and health have been laid bare by the pitiless demands of a virus, and which calls for a new collective examination of how we think of Me and Us.

REFERENCES

Introduction

1. Redelmeier DA, Tversky A. Discrepancy between medical decisions for individual patients and for groups. *N Engl J Med.* 1990; 322(16): 1162–1164. doi: 10.1056/NEJM199004193221620
2. Garton Ash T. *Free World: America, Europe, and the Surprising Future of the West.* New York, NY: Vintage Books; 2005.
3. Dumitrescu I. Don't get too comfortable. *The New York Review.* May 27, 2021. https://nybooks.com/articles/2021/05/27/eula-biss-dont-get-too-comfortable

Chapter 1

1. Chetty R, Stepner M, Abraham S, et al. The association between income and life expectancy in the United States, 2001–2014. *JAMA.* 2016; 315(16): 1750–1766. doi: 10.1001/jama.2016.4226
2. Olshansky SJ, Barnes BA, Cassel C. In search of Methuselah: Estimating the upper limits of human longevity. *Science.* 1990; 250: 634–640. doi: 10.1126/science.2237414
3. Avendano M, Glymour MM, Banks J, Mackenbach JP. Health disadvantage in US adults aged 50 to 74 years: A comparison of the health of rich and poor Americans with that of Europeans. *Am J Public Health.* 2009; 99(3): 540–548. doi: 10.2105/AJPH.2008.139469
4. Kelley AC. The "International Human Suffering Index": Reconsideration of the evidence. *Population and Development Review.* 1989; 15(4): 731–737. doi: 10.2307/1972597

Chapter 2

1. Stein MD, Galea S. *Pained: Uncomfortable Conversations About the Public's Health.* New York, NY: Oxford University Press; 2020.

2. Slopen N, Fitzmaurice GM, Williams DR, Gilman SE. Common patterns of violence experiences and depression and anxiety among adolescents. *Soc Psychiatry Psychiatr Epidemiol.* 2012; 47(10): 1591–1605. doi: 10.1007/s00127-011-0466-5

3. McDonald CC, Richmond TR. The relationship between community violence exposure and mental health symptoms in urban adolescents. *J Psychiatr Ment Health Nurs.* 2008; 15: 833–849. doi: 10.1111/j.1365-2850.2008.01321.x

4. Hanna-Attisha M. *What the Eyes Don't See: A Story of Crisis, Resistance and Hope in an American City.* New York, NY: One World; 2018.

5. Solnit R. *Hope in the Dark: Untold Histories, Wild Possibilities.* Chicago, IL: Haymarket; 2016.

6. Chait J. Tucker Carlson thinks lockdowns have nothing to do with flattening the curve. *Intelligencer.* April 28, 2020. https://nymag.com/intelligencer/2020/04/tucker-carlson-lockdowns-tony-fauci-coronavirus.html

7. Rose G. Sick individuals and sick populations. *Int J Epidemiol.* 2001; 30(3): 427–432. doi: 10.1093/ije/30.3.427

Chapter 3

1. United States v. Shinnick, 219 F. Supp. 789 (1963).

2. Rich M. "We're in a Petri dish": How a coronavirus ravaged a cruise ship. *The New York Times.* February 22, 2020. https://www.nytimes.com/2020/02/22/world/asia/coronavirus-japan-cruise-ship.html

3. Moriarty LF, Plucinski MM, Marston BJ, et al. Public health responses to COVID-19 outbreaks on cruise ships—worldwide, February–March 2020. *MMWR Morb Mortal Wkly Rep.* 2020; 67(12): 347–352. doi: 10.15585/mmwr.mm6912e3

4. Kamal R. How does U.S. life expectancy compare to other countries? *KFF.* 2019. https://www.healthsystemtracker.org/chart-collection/u-s-life-expectancy-compare-countries/#item-start

5. Chetty R, Stepner M, Abraham S, et al. The association between income and life expectancy in the United States, 2001–2014. *JAMA.* 2016; 315(16): 1750–1766. doi: 10.1001/jama.2016.4226

6. Cullen MR, Cummins C, Fuchs VR. Geographic and racial variation in premature mortality in the U.S.: Analyzing the disparities. *PLOS One.* 2012; 7(4): e32930. doi: 10.1371/journal.pone.0032930

7. Cutler DM, Glaeser EL, Vigdor JL. *The Rise and Decline of the American Ghetto* [Working Paper 5881]. Cambridge, MA: National Bureau of Economic Research; January 1997. doi: 10.3386/w5881

Chapter 4

1. Adult obesity facts. Centers for Disease Control and Prevention. June 7, 2021. https://www.cdc.gov/obesity/data/adult.html
2. Fisher ES, Wennberg DE, Stukel TA, et al. The implications of regional variations in Medicare spending. Part 1: The content, quality, and accessibility of care. *Ann Intern Med.* 2003; 138(4): 273–287.
3. Sun LH. CDC to cut by 80 percent efforts to prevent global disease outbreak. *The Washington Post.* February 1, 2018. https://www.washingtonpost.com/news/to-your-health/wp/2018/02/01/cdc-to-cut-by-80-percent-efforts-to-prevent-global-disease-outbreak
4. The impact of chronic underfunding on America's public health system: Trends, risks, and recommendations, 2021. Trust for America's Health. May 7, 2021. https://www.tfah.org/report-details/pandemic-proved-underinvesting-in-public-health-lives-livelihoods-risk
5. DeSalvo K, Levi J, Hoagland B, Parekh A. Developing a financing system to support public health infrastructure. Public Health Leadership Forum. n.d. https://www.resolve.ngo/docs/phlf_developingafinancingsystemtosupportpublichealth636869439688663025.pdf
6. Fee E, Brown TM. The unfulfilled promise of public health: Déjà vu all over again. *Health Affairs.* 2002; 21(6): 31–43. doi: 10.1377/hlthaff.21.6.31
7. Starr P. *The Social Transformation of American Medicine: The Rise of a Sovereign Profession and the Making of a Vast Industry.* New York, NY: Basic Books; 2017.
8. Frieden T. Putting a stake through the heart of public health's Eeyore complex. *Health Affairs.* April 27, 2020. doi: 10.1377/hblog20200425.195884
9. National health expenditure data: Historical. Centers for Medicare & Medicaid Services. December 16, 2020. https://www.cms.gov/Research-Statistics-Data-and-Systems/Statistics-Trends-and-Reports/NationalHealthExpendData/NationalHealthAccountsHistorical
10. The master settlement agreement: An overview. Public Health Law Center. January 2019. https://www.publichealthlawcenter.org/sites/default/files/resources/MSA-Overview-2019.pdf
11. Masters R, Anwar E, Collins B, Cookson R, Capewell S. Return on investment of public health interventions: A systematic review. *J Epidemiol Community Health.* 2017; 71: 827–834. doi: 10.1136/jech-2016-208141

12. Tan S, Fraser A, McHugh N, Warner ME. Widening perspectives on social impact bonds. *J Econ Policy Reform*. 2019; 24(1): 1–10. doi: 10.1080/17487870.2019.1568249

13. Milner J, Poethig EC, Roman J, Walsh K. Putting evidence first: Learning from the Rikers Island social impact bond. Urban Institute. July 5, 2015. https://www.urban.org/urban-wire/putting-evidence-first-learning-rikers-island-social-impact-bond

Chapter 5

1. Yellman M, Peterson C, McCoy MA, et al. Preventing deaths and injuries from house fires: A cost–benefit analysis of a community-based smoke alarm installation programme. *Inj Prev*. 2018; 24: 12–18. doi: 10.1136/injuryprev-2016-042247

2. Richter ED, Barach P, Ben-Michael E, Berman T. Death and injury from motor vehicle crashes: A public health failure, not an achievement. *Inj Prev*. 2001; 7: 176–178. doi: 10.1136/ip.7.3.176

3. Richter ED, Barach P, Berman T, Ben-David G, Weinberger Z. Extending the boundaries of the Declaration of Helsinki: A case study of an unethical experiment in a non-medical setting. *J Med Ethics*. 2001; 27(2): 126–129. doi: 10.1136/jme.27.2.126

4. Joksch HC. Velocity change and fatality risk in a crash: A rule of thumb. *Accid Anal Prev*. 1993; 25(1): 103–104. doi: 10.1016/0001-4575(93)90102-3

Chapter 7

1. Pollan M. The sickness in our food supply. *The New York Review*. June 11, 2020. https://nybooks.com/articles/2020/06/11/covid-19-sickness-food-supply

2. Centers for Disease Control and Prevention. Ten great public health achievements—United States, 1900–1999. *MMWR Morb Mortal Wkly Rep*. 1999; 48(12): 241–243. PMID: 10220250

3. Rosen G. *A History of Public Health*. Baltimore, MD: Johns Hopkins University Press; 2015.

4. Gopnik A. *A Thousand Small Sanities*. New York, NY: Basic Books; 2019.

Chapter 8

1. Klinenberg E. *Heat Wave: A Social Autopsy of Disaster in Chicago*. Chicago, IL: University of Chicago Press; 2003.
2. Johnson SB. *The Ghost Map*. New York, NY: Riverhead; 2006.

Part 2

1. Hardin G. The tragedy of the commons: The population problem has no technical solution; it requires a fundamental extension in morality. *Science*. 1968; 162(3859): 1243–1248. doi: 10.1126/science.162.3859.1243
2. Aristotle. *Politics: Book Two*. Oxford, UK: Clarendon; 1905.
3. Duhigg C. Millions in U.S. drink dirty water, records show. *The New York Times*. December 7, 2009. https://www.nytimes.com/2009/12/08/business/energy-environment/08water.html
4. Galea S. It is time to think differently about health. *Fortune*. May 8, 2019. https://fortune.com/2019/05/08/healthcare-public-good
5. U.S. National Action Plan for Combating Antibiotic-Resistant Bacteria. Centers for Disease Control and Prevention. October 2020. https://www.cdc.gov/drugresistance/us-activities/national-action-plan.html
6. McCloskey E. Is $1 enough for viral hepatitis prevention? NASTAD. July 27, 2014. https://www.nastad.org/blog/1-enough-viral-hepatitis-prevention
7. Developing mechanisms for billing. Centers for Disease Control and Prevention. November 15, 2019. https://www.cdc.gov/vaccines/programs/billables-project/billing.html
8. Fact sheet: Biden–Harris administration to invest $7 billion from American Rescue Plan to hire and train public health workers in response to COVID-19. The White House. May 13, 2021. https://www.whitehouse.gov/briefing-room/statements-releases/2021/05/13/fact-sheet-biden-harris-administration-to-invest-7-billion-from-american-rescue-plan-to-hire-and-train-public-health-workers-in-response-to-covid-19
9. Fee E, Brown TM. The unfulfilled promise of public health: Déjà vu all over again. *Health Affairs*. 2002; 21(6): 31–43. doi: 10.1377/hlthaff.21.6.31
10. Davies SC, Pearson-Stuttard J. *Whose Health Is It, Anyway?* New York, NY: Oxford University Press; 2021: 14.
11. County health rankings model. University of Wisconsin Population Health Institute. March 29, 2016. https://www.countyhealthrankings.org/resources/county-health-rankings-model

12. Himmelstein DU, Woolhandler S. Public health's falling share of US health spending. *Am J Public Health.* 2016; 106(1): 56–57. doi: 10.2105/AJPH.2015.302908

13. Bridgeland J, Orszag P. Can government play moneyball? *The Atlantic.* 2013. https://www.theatlantic.com/magazine/archive/2013/07/can-government-play-moneyball/309389

14. Hendren N, Sprung-Keyser B. A unified welfare analysis of government policies. *Q J Econ.* 2020; 135(3): 1209–1318. doi: 10.1093/qje/qjaa006

15. Chetty R, Hendren N, Katz LF. The effects of exposure to better neighborhoods on children: New evidence from the Moving to Opportunity experiment. *Am Econ Rev.* 2016; 106(4): 855–902. doi: 10.1257/aer.20150572

16. Chetty R, Friedman JN, Hendren N, Jones MR, Porter SR. *The Opportunity Atlas: Mapping the Childhood Roots of Social Mobility* [Working Paper 25147]. Cambridge, MA: National Bureau of Economic Research; 2018. doi: 10.3386/w25147

17. Bayer R, Galea S. Public health in the precision-medicine era. *N Engl J Med.* 2015; 373: 499–501. doi: 10.1056/NEJMp1506241

18. Moses H, Dorsey ER, Matheson DHM, Thier SO. Financial anatomy of biomedical research. *JAMA.* 2005; 294(11): 1333–1342. doi: 10.1001/jama.294.11.1333

19. Lyu W, Wehby GL. Community use of face masks and COVID-19: Evidence from a natural experiment of state mandates in the US. *Health Affairs.* 2020; 39(8): 1419–1425. doi: 10.1377/hlthaff.2020.00818

20. Wilson RT, Troisi CL, Gary-Webb TL. A deficit of more than 250,000 public health workers is no way to fight Covid-19. *Stat News.* April 5, 2020. https://www.statnews.com/2020/04/05/deficit-public-health-workers-no-way-to-fight-covid-19

21. Beitsch LM, Castrucci BC, Dilley A, et al. From patchwork to package: Implementing foundational capabilities for state and local health departments. *Am J Public Health.* 2015; 105: e7–e10. doi: 10.2105/AJPH.2014.302369

INDEX

For the benefit of digital users, indexed terms that span two pages (e.g., 52–53) may, on occasion, appear on only one of those pages.